NUTRITION and Type 2 DIABETES

NUTRITION
and Type 2
DIABETES
Etiology and Prevention

Edited by
Mark A. Pereira

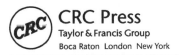

CRC Press
Taylor & Francis Group
Boca Raton London New York

CRC Press is an imprint of the
Taylor & Francis Group, an **informa** business

CRC Press
Taylor & Francis Group
6000 Broken Sound Parkway NW, Suite 300
Boca Raton, FL 33487-2742

First issued in paperback 2019

ISBN-13: 978-1-4398-5032-9 (hbk)
ISBN-13: 978-0-367-37957-5 (pbk)

Library of Congress Cataloging-in-Publication Data

Nutrition and type 2 diabetes : etiology and prevention / editor, Mark A. Pereira.
  p. ; cm.
  Includes bibliographical references and index.
  ISBN 978-1-4398-5032-9 (hardcover : alk. paper)
  I. Pereira, Mark A.
  [DNLM: 1. Diabetes Mellitus, Type 2--epidemiology. 2. Clinical Trials as Topic.
3. Cohort Studies. 4. Diabetes Mellitus, Type 2--etiology. 5. Nutritional Physiological Phenomena. WK 810]

  RC662.2
  616.4'6240654--dc23   2013010840

Visit the Taylor & Francis Web site at
http://www.taylorandfrancis.com

and the CRC Press Web site at
http://www.crcpress.com

Contents

CONTENTS

Preface

Over a relatively short period of time, the last few decades, type 2 diabetes has emerged as a leading threat to global health. It is likely no coincidence that there is considerable overlap in the obesity and diabetes trends of the last few decades in most developed and now also developing regions of the world. The underpinnings for type 2 diabetes etiology, as with obesity, are found in lifestyles, particularly in the dietary and physical activity patterns. Scientists and practitioners continue to struggle in understanding the complexities of dietary composition in terms of optimal approaches for preventing and managing type 2 diabetes. This issue is much more than a matter of energy balance and obesity but, importantly, it is a matter of where the energy comes from, and the context of the diet in terms of preparation and composition. The mediating/mechanistic role of obesity and body composition are appropriately covered throughout the text when necessary. It is my hope that this book will benefit medical and public health scientists, graduate students, dietitians, physicians, and other research- and practice-based health professionals interested in improving their grasp of the scientific evidence on the etiology and epidemiology of type 2 diabetes, the foundation upon which prevention efforts should reside. Throughout, you will learn fundamental nutritional principals applied to the pathophysiology of type 2 diabetes as well as applied behavioral studies on nutrition and diabetes in each content area. The authors are all leading and prolific researchers in the field, each with unique perspectives and important contributions. They have my gratitude for setting aside time that could have been well spent in other endeavors, in order to introduce us to many important principles and lessons in this rapidly evolving field.

Mark Pereira
Minneapolis, Minn.

Editor

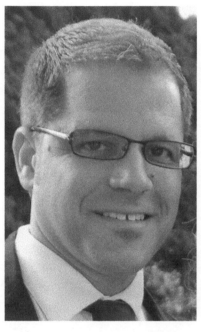

Mark Pereira earned his Ph.D. in Epidemiology from the University of Pittsburgh. From 1996-1999 he was an NIH/National Heart, Lung, and Blood Institute Postdoctoral Fellow in Cardiovascular Epidemiology at the University of Minnesota. Dr. Pereira was a Research Associate at Children's Hospital, Boston and a faculty member of the Department of Pediatrics, Harvard Medical School from 1999-2003. Since 2003 he has been on faculty in the Division of Epidemiology & Community Health in the School of Public Health at the University of Minnesota, Minneapolis, where he is currently an Associate Professor and Program Director of Public Health Nutrition. In 2012 he received the *Outstanding Faculty Award* from the Council of Graduate Students of the University of Minnesota. His research focuses on non-communicable disease etiology and epidemiology, with particular emphasis on the pathways between environmental/lifestyle factors and chronic disease risk, with a special focus on type 2 diabetes. Dr. Pereira's research is trans-disciplinary and spans from small controlled trials to large-scale epidemiologic cohort studies, including international cohort studies. His research is primarily funded by the National Institutes of Health, and has also been funded by the American Heart Association and a variety of other sources. He currently serves as the principal investigator on a large five-year grant funded by the National Institute of Diabetes and Digestive and Kidney Diseases to examine environmental and genetic determinants of type 2 diabetes in the Singapore Chinese

Health Study. In the classroom Dr. Pereira teaches graduate courses in public health nutrition and writing research grant applications. His publication record includes over 100 peer-reviewed scientific journal articles, reviews, editorials, and book chapters.

Mark A. Pereira, PhD
April, 2013

Contributors

Frank B. Hu, MD, ScD
Harvard University

Lawrence de Koning, PhD
University of Calgary
Calgary, Alberta, Canada

Simin Liu, MD, ScD
Brown University

Vasanti S. Malik, ScD
Harvard University

Noel T. Mueller, MPH
University of Minnesota

Andrew O. Odegaard, PhD
University of Minnesota

Mark A. Pereira, PhD
University of Minnesota

Yan Song, MD, MS
University of Southern California,
Los Angeles

Yiqing Song, MD, ScD
Brigham and Women's Hospital,
Harvard Medical School

chapter one

Introduction

Mark A. Pereira, PhD
University of Minnesota

Contents

Type 2 diabetes: A pandemic at full bore

Type 2 diabetes (T2D), typically resulting from a combination of resistance to insulin in the peripheral tissues, as well as relative insulin deficiency, has emerged over the past two decades as a major global health problem. T2D is a common and very costly chronic disease, which increases risk for morbidity and mortality through a plethora of micro- and macro-vascular diseases resulting from the toxicity of hyperglycemia as well as highly common cardiovascular maladies that typically coincide with T2D, including dyslipidemia and hypertension (Engelgau, Geiss et al. 2004). T2D is thus one of the leading consumers of healthcare costs (Engelgau, Geiss et al. 2004; Hossain, Kawar et al. 2007). Rates are increasing through-out the developed and developing world, related closely to "westerniza-tion," sedentary lifestyle, and the associated changes in the food supply in terms of availability, abundance, and composition. The International Diabetes Federation has estimated the number of persons living with dia-betes around the globe, as shown in Figure 1.1, contrasting the number of cases in the year 2000 to the projected numbers for the year 2030 (Wild, Roglic et al. 2004; Hossain, Kawar et al. 2007).

When one considers the nature of the epidemiologic transition from scarcity and infection to abundance and noncommunicable disease, it becomes understandable that as developing populations transition in the

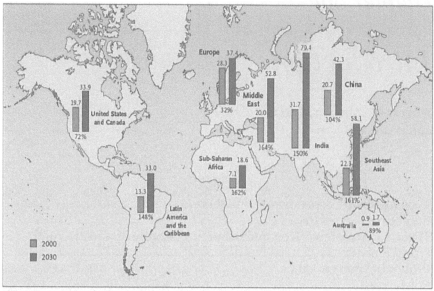

Millions of Cases of Diabetes in 2000 and Projections for 2030, with Projected Percent Changes.
Data are from Wild and Roglic, 2004.   N ENGL J MED 356;3 www.nejm.org JANUARY 18, 2007

Figure 1.1 The diabetes pandemic.

face of globalization and westernization, T2D rates typically begin to rise, along with increases in overweight and obesity, cardiovascular diseases, and certain cancers (Omran 1971; Yoon 2006; Hossain, Kawar et al. 2007; WHO 2008). The World Health Organization and International Diabetes Federation have recognized T2D as a pressing pandemic (IDI 2003; 2004). Based on projections from existing surveillance systems around the globe, the number of people with diabetes is expected to increase from 194 million in the year 2003 to 333 million by the year 2025, with the crude prevalence rate expected to increase by 20% (IDI 2003). Unfortunately, rates and absolute numbers of cases of T2D are expected to increase the most in many developing regions, particularly throughout parts of Asia, that may be the least equipped to deal with such a public health crisis (Yoon 2006). Due to the increases in prevalence and the increasing size of the populations in these areas, T2D cases are expected to increase in Southeast Asia from 39 million to 82 million between the years 2003 and 2025 (Yoon 2006). In Singapore, the prevalence of diabetes is expected to increase from 12.3% in 2003 to 19.5% in 2025, when it will rank as the third highest in the world behind Nauru (33% expected) and the United Arab Emirates (24.5% expected) (Yoon 2006).

Etiological perspectives

Although age, ethnicity, and, to some substantial yet still unclear extent, genetics play important roles in T2D etiology, it is the modifiable risk factors that are most telling. Obesity, relatively high stores of body fat, is a formidable predictor of T2D at the population level, but the association between obesity and diabetes risk is not robust ecologically, between populations (Yoon 2006). Indeed, as can be observed from the data in Figure 1.1, South/Southeast Asia is a hotbed for T2D despite this region having much lower rates of obesity than most European countries and much of the west, including the United States (Yoon 2006; Hossain, Kawar et al. 2007). Furthermore, among those with similar levels of total body fat, or relative body weight, it is difficult to predict who will and who will not go on to develop the disease (St-Onge, Janssen et al. 2004; Thamer, Machann et al. 2004; Pereira, Kottke et al. 2009). This difficulty is likely due to the heterogeneity of genetics, fitness, body composition, physical activity, dietary habits, and many interactions among all of these factors. We must turn our attention to clinical studies and epidemiological cohort studies in order to advance our understanding of the causal pathological agents of T2D within and across populations. Scientific discovery from such observational and experimental work will be critical toward the ultimate goal of improving our ability to screen, risk stratify, prevent, and treat T2D, especially in parts of the developing world with high disease rates and compromised healthcare systems.

As with physical activity, dietary modification, through a variety of means, is known to be very important in controlling blood sugar, and therefore, potentially effecting T2D risk (Hu, vanDam et al. 2001; Pereira, Kottke et al. 2009). In addition to direct effects on blood sugar control, dietary modification has the potential to change body composition, particularly the size of the fat depots and possibly the partitioning of fat between the visceral versus subcutaneous depots (Pereira, Kottke et al. 2009; Stanhope 2009; Maersk, Belza et al. 2012; Odegaard, Choh et al. 2012). Indeed, several long-term behavioral intervention studies of diet and exercise interventions have consistently demonstrated the efficacy of diet and exercise in the primary prevention of T2D risk (Pan, Li et al. 1997; Tuomilehto, Lindstrom et al. 2001; Knowler, Barrett-Connor et al. 2002). Despite varying degrees of weight loss, usually a modest amount of 2% to 6% across these studies, and the cultural and ethnic variations across the studies, the results on preventing diabetes through lifestyle are remarkably consistent. A statistically significant, and certainly clinically significant, 30% to 60% reduction in the risk of diabetes was reported across the studies (Pan, Li et al. 1997; Tuomilehto, Lindstrom et al. 2001; Knowler, Barrett-Connor et al. 2002). Two of the studies combined diet and exercise in the intervention to maximize efficacy and use resources efficiently

(Tuomilehto, Lindstrom et al. 2001; Knowler, Barrett-Connor et al. 2002). However, one interesting exception was the first intervention study on diabetes prevention by lifestyle—The Da Qing Study in Chinese adults (Pan, Li et al. 1997). In the Da Qing Study, a factorial parallel design was used, with participants, lean and overweight adults with glucose intolerance but not frank diabetes, randomized to one of four groups: Control, Nutrition intervention, Exercise intervention, or Nutrition + Exercise intervention. Interestingly, all three intervention groups experienced a significant reduction in diabetes risk compared to the control group, but the combined Nutrition + Exercise group did not experience a larger decrease in risk, perhaps due to the difficulty of adhering to two interventions simultaneously. There are two further aspects of this study that are important to describe. The first is that the efficacy of these interventions appeared to be equivalent for both the lean as well as the overweight participants. Although the absolute rates of diabetes were higher for the overweight, the relative risk of incident diabetes over the course of the study declined to a similar extent for the overweight and the lean, compared to those in the control group. This observation supports a wealth of metabolic studies in animals and humans supporting direct effects of diet and exercise on improving glucose control independent of body composition or any changes in body composition (Kriska, Blair et al. 1994; Pereira, Kottke et al. 2009). The second important aspect of the Da-Qing Trial is its profound impact on long-term diabetes risk. Li et al. (2008) recently reported the 20-year follow-up diabetes rates of the original Da-Qing Trial participants. As shown in Figure 1.2, those randomized to the intervention arms of the study experienced a 51% reduction in diabetes risk, compared to the control group, at 6 years. The very long-term 20-year follow-up demonstrated a sustained effect of the intervention, with a highly statistically significant risk reduction of 43%. T2D is preventable, by reasonable lifestyle changes, in lean and overweight adults. The key is likely to intervene before it is too late, as T2D goes undiagnosed for years in many cases, and once the pancreas looses a critical mass of beta cells, insulin deficiency and in all likelihood irreversible diabetes will ensue.

Theoretical framework on understanding the role of nutrition and type 2 diabetes

Despite the well-accepted importance of nutrition and dietary behavior in the etiology of T2D and in its primary prevention, scientists and practitioners continue to struggle, as they do with diet and obesity, in understanding the specific aspects of the diet that may directly, or even indirectly, impact diabetes risk. An enormous wealth of literature has been published on this topic. These studies include numerous large epidemiologic

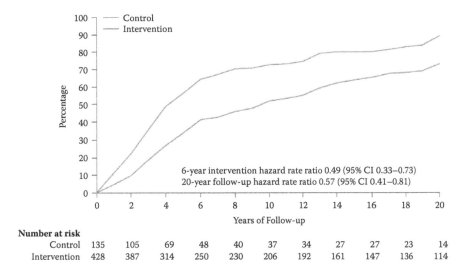

Figure 1.2 Cumulative incidence of diabetes mellitus during follow-up in China Da Qing Diabetes Prevention Outcome Study. (From Li et al. (2008), *Lancet* 2008; 371: 1783–89.)

cohort studies, as well as carefully conducted randomized trials. The goal of the book is to examine, with methodological rigor, various perspectives on diet and T2D, including specific nutrients, foods, and overall dietary patterns (from *"soup to nuts"*). Therefore, this book does not discuss T2D management/treatment, as this clinical context has been covered extensively elsewhere (DeFronzo, Ferrannini et al. 2004). The goal here is to cover etiology and epidemiology, and focus primarily on the human literature (with some animal data in supportive/complimentary form only when necessary or for background sections). Along those lines, one area of research that remains relatively sparse is experimental studies in humans from which we are able to isolate specific dietary effects independent of other confounding factors within those trials, for example, multiple dietary changes, body composition changes, and physical activity. The mediating/mechanistic role of obesity and body composition will be covered throughout the book whenever appropriate. However, alterations in body composition, amounts and types of body fat and skeletal muscle, is primarily viewed as a mediating or modifying factor through which dietary composition may exert its effects on blood glucose control. Obesity etiology, epidemiology, prevention, and treatment has been well covered in several other textbooks (Bray and Bouchard 2004a; Bray and Bouchard 2004a; Hu 2008). Figure 1.3 depicts a general/simplistic theoretical framework through which dietary and nutritional factors, as well as physical activity, may impact risk for T2D.

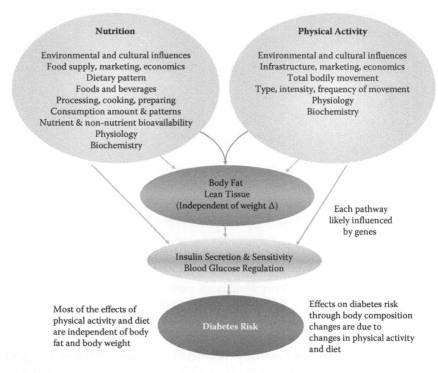

Figure 1.3 Pathways through which lifestyle may impact type 2 diabetes risk.

The complicated etiology of T2D from the perspective of the life course is depicted in Figure 1.4. Although the role of genetics is thought to be critical, the impact of genes is likely modified to a significant degree through the many environmental and lifestyle factors that are known to predict diabetes risk. As is also the case for obesity, the discovery of genetic lesions for T2D to date has been quite modest [ref]. Indeed, the escalating prevalence of obesity globally, and the pandemic of T2D following closely behind, is telling with respect to the limited application genetics information is likely to yield in primary and secondary prevention. On the other hand, tremendous progress has been made on the lifestyle/environmental side of the equation for diabetes prevention, with the dietary and nutritional components being dissected throughout this book. As shown in Figure 1.4, there are a number of opportunities throughout the life course to capitalize on primary and secondary prevention of T2D. The questions that need to be considered, in light of the complexity of T2D etiology, include the following.

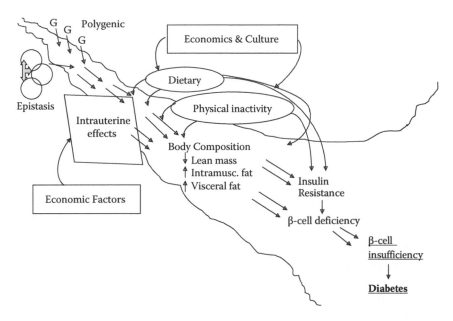

Figure 1.4 The complexity of type 2 diabetes etiology through the life course.

1. When should we intervene? We could and arguably should intervene in utero through maternal lifestyle interventions that reduce the risk of chronic disease in the present and future for mother and child.
2. What population subgroup should be a priority for intervention, if any?
3. What should be the intervention targets and methods—diet, exercise, body composition, pharmacological agents, or some combination?
4. At what levels of the socioecological framework should interventions or policies be implemented—the individual, family, community, school, worksite, healthcare system, etc.?

The goal of this book is to provide a review of the science on the potential impact of many, but certainly not all, components of dietary behavior and nutritional properties on etiology and risk for T2D. Mastery of this literature is essential to avoid naïve approaches that may do more harm than good in addressing the above questions that are essential to public health progress in this area.

Primordial prevention

In the 1970s, before what some refer to as the "obesity epidemic" of the last three decades, the Dr. Toma Strasser,* Former Chief Officer of the Cardiovascular Division of the World Health Organization as well as an investigator of the former Yugoslavian Segment of the Seven Countries Study, was concerned about the potential for a cardiovascular disease pandemic, which often coincides with T2D due to very common etiologic pathways and risk factors. At that time, Strasser coined the term "primordial prevention," proposing the only sure solution to preventing global epidemics is a focus on preventing the risk factors themselves. In his words: "*While the epidemic of (cardiovascular) risk factors has pervaded the consumer societies, it still has not reached the majority of the developing world. Real grassroot prevention should start by preserving entire risk factor epidemics. Here lies the possibility of averting one of tomorrow's world health problems. For expressing this important concept, I wish to propose the term of protoprophylaxis, or primordial prevention*" (Strasser, 1978). Strasser's *primordial prevention* is a unifying theme of this book. We must take it more seriously because the fate of future generations is still in our control.

What ensues in the following chapters is a rigorous, comprehensive description and evaluation of the central research to date, primarily in humans, on the macronutrients and their subclasses, micronutrients, foods, beverages, and overall dietary patterns with respect to the risk of T2D. Within the chapters on nutrients, important references and translations are made to the food and food-group sources of those nutrients. This strategy is highly relevant and important, as the winds in the field of nutritional epidemiology have gradually shifted over recent years, extending from a central focus on isolated components of the diet, primarily nutrients ("magic bullets"), toward a more comprehensive and applicable perspective on the whole foods and the interactions between foods and their components across the whole diet. This concept of "food synergy" was introduced and emphasized by David R. Jacobs, Jr. and colleagues, who pioneered epidemiologic studies of whole grains (see Chapter 2) that had a major influence on the evolving *Dietary Guidelines for Americans* and on certain industry approaches to the formulation and marketing of grain products (Jacobs, Marquart et al. 1998; Jacobs, Pereira et al. 2000; Jacobs and Steffen 2003; Jacobs 2007; Jacobs 2009 et al.). The depth and breadth of this book includes aspects of the "food synergy" model for understanding the complicated pathways between nutrition, dietary habits, and risk for T2D.

* For more on Strasser and his peers, visit Dr. Henry Blackburn's *History of Cardiovascular Epidemiology* at http://www.epi.umn.edu/cvdepi/index.html.

References

Bray, G. A. and C. Bouchard, Eds. (2004). *Handbook of Obesity: Clinical Applications.* New York, Marcel Dekker.

DeFronzo, R. A., E. Ferrannini et al., Eds. (2004). *International Textbook of Diabetes Mellitus*, Wiley.

Engelgau, M. M., L. S. Geiss et al. (2004). "The evolving diabetes burden in the United States." *Ann Intern Med* **140**(11): 945–950.

Hossain, P., B. Kawar et al. (2007). "Obesity and diabetes in the developing world— A growing challenge." *N Engl J Med* **356**(3): 213–215.

Hu, F. B. (2008). *Obesity Epidemiology.* New York, Oxford University Press.

Hu, F. B., R. M. van Dam, et al. (2001). "Diet and risk of Type II diabetes: The role of types of fat and carbohydrate." *Diabetologia* **44**(7): 805–817.

IDI (2003). Diabetes Atlas Summary of the International Diabetes Federation. Brussels, Belgium, International Diabetes Federation: 58.

Jacobs, D. R., Jr., L. Marquart, et al. (1998). "Whole-grain intake and cancer: An expanded review and meta-analysis." *Nutr Cancer* **30**(2): 85–96.

Jacobs, D. R., Jr. and L. M. Steffen (2003). "Nutrients, foods, and dietary patterns as exposures in research: A framework for food synergy." *Am J Clin Nutr* **78**(3 suppl.): 508S–513S.

Jacobs, D. R., Jr., M. D. Gross, and L. C. Tapsell (2009). "Food synergy: An operational concept for understanding nutrition." *Am J Clin Nutr* **89** (suppl.): 1S–6S.

Jacobs, D. R., Jr., and L. C. Tapsell (2007). "Food, not nutrients, is the fundamental unit in nutrition." *Nutr Rev* **65**(10): 439–450.

Jacobs, D. R., M. Pereira et al. (2000). "Defining the impact of whole grain intake on chronic desease." *Cereal Foods World* **45**: 51–53.

Knowler, W. C., E. Barrett-Connor et al. (2002). "Reduction in the incidence of type 2 diabetes with lifestyle intervention or metformin." *N Engl J Med* **346**(6): 393–403.

Kriska, A. M., S. N. Blair et al. (1994). "The potential role of physical activity in the prevention of non-insulin-dependent diabetes mellitus: The epidemiological evidence." *Exerc Sport Sci Rev* **22**: 121–143.

Maersk, M., A. Belza et al. (2012). "Sucrose-sweetened beverages increase fat storage in the liver, muscle, and visceral fat depot: a 6-mo randomized intervention study." *Am J Clin Nutr* **95**(2): 283–289.

Li, G., P. Zhang et al. (2008). "The long-term effects of lifestyle interventions to prevent diabetes in the China Da Qing Diabetes Study: a 20-year follow-up study. *Lancet* **371**(9626): 1783–1789.

Odegaard, A. O., A. C. Choh et al. (2012). "Sugar-sweetened and diet beverages in relation to visceral adipose tissue." *Obesity (Silver Spring)* **20**(3): 689–691.

Omran, A. (1971). "The epidemiologic transition. A theory of the epidemiology of population change." *The Milbank Memorial Fund Quarterly* **49**(4): 509–538.

Pan, X. R., G. W. Li, et al. (1997). "Effects of diet and exercise in preventing NIDDM in people with impaired glucose tolerance: The Da Qing IGT and Diabetes Study." *Diabetes Care* **20**(4): 537–544.

Pereira, M. A., T. E. Kottke et al. (2009). "Preventing and managing cardiometabolic risk: The logic for intervention." *Int J Environ Res Public Health* **6**(10): 2568–2584.

St-Onge, M. P., I. Janssen et al. (2004). "Metabolic syndrome in normal-weight Americans: New definition of the metabolically obese, normal-weight individual." *Diabetes Care* **27**(9): 2222–2228.

Stanhope, K. L., J. M. Schwarz, N. L. Keim, S. C. Griffen, A. A. Bremer, J. L. Graham, B. Hatcher, C. L. Cox, A. Dyachenko, W. Zhang, J. P. McGahan, A. Seibert, R. M. Krauss, S. Chiu, E. J. Schaefer, M. Ai, S. Otokozawa, K. Nakajima, T. Nakano, C. Beysen, M. K. Hellerstein, L. Berglund, and P. J. Havel (2009). "Consuming fructose-sweetened, not glucose-sweetened, beverages increases visceral adiposity and lipids and decreases insulin sensitivity in overweight/obese humans." *J Clin Invest* **119**(5): 1322–1334.

Strasser, "Reflections on cardiovascular diseases." *Interdisciplinary Science Review* **3**:225–30.

Thamer, C., J. Machann et al. (2004). "Intrahepatic lipids are predicted by visceral adipose tissue mass in healthy subjects." *Diabetes Care* **27**(11): 2726–2729.

Tuomilehto, J., J. Lindstrom et al. (2001). "Prevention of type 2 diabetes mellitus by changes in lifestyle among subjects with impaired glucose tolerance." *N Engl J Med* **344**(18): 1343–1350.

WHO (2008). The global burden of disease: 2004 update. Geneva, World Health Organization.

Wild, S., G. Roglic et al. (2004). "Global prevalence of diabetes: Estimates for the year 2000 and projections for 2030." *Diabetes Care* **27**(5): 1047–1053.

Yoon, K. H., Lee. J. H., Kim, J. W., Cho, J. H., Choi, Y. H., Ko, S. H., Zimmet, P., and Son, H. Y. (2006). "Epidemic obesity and type 2 diabetes in Asia." *Lancet* **368**(9548): 1681–1688.

chapter two

Dietary carbohydrates and type 2 diabetes

Lawrence de Koning, PhD,* Vasanti S. Malik, ScD,* and Frank B. Hu, MD, ScD

Contents

* Contributed equally to this document.

Introduction

Carbohydrates are macromolecules that are named for their constituent components of carbon, hydrogen, and oxygen (hydrate). Along with fat and protein, carbohydrates are one of three major nutrients that can be metabolized into energy. On average, carbohydrates provide 4 kcal of food energy per gram and the majority of total energy in the human diet.

Carbohydrates are especially important to type 2 diabetes because it is a disease of carbohydrate metabolism, and is defined by a sustained elevation of blood glucose. The major determinant of blood glucose is dietary carbohydrate.

Types of carbohydrates

Carbohydrates are often classified by their molecular structure, although this may have little to do with their relationship with health. Monosaccharides or "simple sugars," are the simplest form of carbohydrates. Monosaccharides have at least three carbons, a single carbonyl group, and hydroxyl groups on every carbon atom. Monosaccharides are further defined as to whether their carbonyl group is an aldehyde (aldose) or ketone (ketose). Carbohydrates that are the most relevant to energy metabolism and diabetes risk contain 6 carbons. These are called aldo or keto-hexoses, the most important of which are glucose and fructose. Glucose is the main source of energy for the brain, intestinal cells and red blood cells, and is stored as glycogen in liver and muscle, and as fat in adipose tissue. Fructose, or fruit sugar, has an intensely sweet flavor and must be converted to glyceraldehyde-3-phosphate before it can enter glycolysis to produce ATP (Voet and Voet 2011).

Monosaccharides can be linked together via a glycosidic bond to form larger molecules. The union of two monosaccharides is called a *disaccharide*, whereas a long polymer of monosaccharides is called a *polysaccharide*. Glycosidic bonds are covalent bonds between monosaccharides, and are formed by combining one sugar molecule's hydroxyl group and another's hydrogen to liberate a water molecule. Disaccharides, which are also considered sugars, include sucrose, maltose, and lactose. Sucrose, which is known as *table sugar*, is formed by the union of glucose and fructose. Lactose is the dominant sugar in milk and is a combination of glucose and galactose. Maltose is simply the combination of two glucose molecules. These sugars have glycosidic bonds with an alpha 1,4 orientation, which can be cleaved by digestive enzymes (e.g., sucrase). That is, the bond between the two sugars is established between the 1st carbon of the first sugar and the 4th carbon of the second sugar in a downward orientation to the plane of the molecule (Voet and Voet 2011).

Starch, or amylose, is a plant polysaccharide consisting of thousands of glucose molecules linked by alpha 1,4 glycosidic bonds (Voet and Voet 2011). As with disaccharides, these molecules can be cleaved by digestive enzymes (e.g., amylase) to form smaller subunits (e.g., maltose). Oligo- or disaccharides are then further broken down to liberate monosaccharides using other enzymes (e.g., alpha-glucosidase). Amylopectin is a branched form of amylose, and is a major source of energy in plants. In this molecule, starch chains are stacked neatly upon each other due to alpha 1,6 glycosidic bonds. These are present at every 20–24 glucose residues, and attach vertically to other alpha 1,4 glucose chains so that each is oriented 180 degrees from each other. This allows the molecule to assume a highly packed structure. Alpha 1-6 glycosidic bonds are broken by digestive enzymes such as alpha dextranase, or debranching enzyme. Glycogen, which is found exclusively in animals, is structurally similar to amylopectin except that branch points occur every 8–12 glucose residues (Voet and Voet 2011).

Dietary fibers are structural polysaccharides found in the cell walls of plants. While they appear similar to starch, they contain beta 1,4 glycosidic bonds that cannot be cleaved by digestive enzymes in vertebrates. However, these bonds can be broken by enzymes in microorganisms that are used by ruminants to provide energy from normally indigestible plant material (Voet and Voet 2011). The most common dietary fiber is cellulose, which makes up 80% of the dry weight of plants. Cellulose is classified as an insoluble fiber because it does not dissolve in water. Other insoluble fibers include lignans and hemicelluloses. Soluble fibers dissolve in water to form a gel, and include pectins, gums, and mucilages. All fibers are partially fermented by gut bacteria to form methane and hydrogen; however, soluble fibers are more completely fermented (Howarth, Saltzman et al. 2001).

Food sources of carbohydrate

Human populations appear to have evolved on a wide variety of diets ranging from those rich in plants (herbivorous) to those that were nearly exclusively animals (carnivorous). The major dietary sources of carbohydrate were fruits, vegetables, tubers, and legumes (Eaton 2006). Fruits such as apples provide mostly sugars (e.g., fructose), soluble fiber, insoluble fiber, and some starch. Vegetables and tubers provide mostly insoluble fiber and starch. Legumes (e.g., peas, beans, lentils) provide starch, soluble fiber, and 20%–25% protein by weight (Whitney and Rolfes 2008). However, protein from legumes is deficient in methionine and therefore must be combined with other protein sources to provide all essential amino acids in the diet (Whitney and Rolfes 2008).

With the development of agriculture and the domestication of cere-als approximately 10,000 years ago, corn, wheat, and rice began to dis-place fruits, vegetables, tubers, and legumes to become the largest dietary sources of carbohydrate. This occurred because cereals are easily cultivated in large quantities, have high energy density, and can be stored for long periods (Eaton and Eaton 2000). Large-scale cultivation of cereals is cred-ited with the rapid increase in human populations (Eaton and Eaton 2000).

Rice (*Oryza* sp.) was domesticated in China, and is one of the most widely consumed cereals in the world (Vaughan, Lu et al. 2008). In the traditional diets of rural China and India, rice provides 70% or more of total calories (Du, Lu et al. 2002). Similar to the tomato and potato, maize/corn (*Zea mays*) was domesticated in Central America (Doebley 2004), and is currently the most widely cultivated cereal in the world (Howarth, Saltzman et al. 2001). This is because a large proportion of maize is pro-duced for livestock feed and biofuels. Wheat (*Triticum* sp.) was domesti-cated in the Middle East (Lev-Yadun, Gopher et al. 2000), and is unique in its protein content, which contains all essential amino acids. The amount of wheat and rice grown in the world is approximately equal (Howarth, Saltzman et al. 2001).

Cereal grains all have the same basic anatomical features (Figure 2.1). The majority of the grain by weight and volume is starch-rich endosperm, which is used as an energy source for the growing plant (Whitney and Rolfes 2008). The embryonic plant, or germ, is high in protein, antioxi-dants, fats, and vitamins. The outer envelope, or bran/husk, is rich in insoluble fiber, but also antioxidants, some vitamins, and minerals such as magnesium and zinc (Whitney and Rolfes 2008).

Although grains are highly nutritious in their unaltered form, they are often mechanically refined and milled to remove bran and germ. This

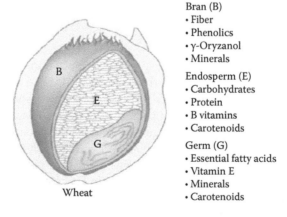

Bran (B)
• Fiber
• Phenolics
• γ-Oryzanol
• Minerals

Endosperm (E)
• Carbohydrates
• Protein
• B vitamins
• Carotenoids

Germ (G)
• Essential fatty acids
• Vitamin E
• Minerals
• Carotenoids

Wheat

Figure 2.1 Anatomy of a whole grain kernel. (Unknown source.)

increases palatability, shelf life, and decreases cooking time. However, refining drastically reduces nutritional content (Food and Agriculture Organization of the United Nations 2009). For example, white flour, which is mostly finely ground and bleached endosperm, has 80% less fiber, 30% less protein, and 10% more calories per gram compared to whole wheat flour (Whitney and Rolfes 2008). With the loss of the bran and germ, refined flour is also stripped of important vitamins and minerals. For example, white flour is 60%–70% lower in thiamine (B1), riboflavin (B2), vitamin B6, magnesium, and zinc compared to whole-wheat flour (Whitney and Rolfes 2008). As part of a public health initiative to reduce the incidence of neural tube defects, B-vitamins are added back to white flour to produce "enriched" flour. Minerals are not commonly added back (Whitney and Rolfes 2008). Further refinement can be performed on ground endosperm to yield concentrated liquid sugar. Cornstarch is processed enzymatically to liberate glucose and fructose that forms the basis of corn syrup (Whitney and Rolfes 2008). High-fructose corn syrup is one of the largest single sources of calories in the Western diet, contributing 8% to the American diet in 2004 (Duffey and Popkin 2008). Total carbohydrate in the diet is the sum of all digestible forms of carbohydrate, which includes refined carbohydrates as liquid- and solid-added sugars, and refined grains such as white bread, potatoes and tubers, whole grains, legumes, fruit, vegetables, and also lactose from dairy.

Trends in carbohydrate intake

In the United States, total carbohydrate consumption decreased from 500 g/d in 1909 to 374 g/d in 1963, which was largely due to decreases in the consumption of whole grains (Gross, Li et al. 2004) [Figure 2.2]. Over this same time period, intake of dietary fiber decreased by nearly 40%. However, since 1963, the consumption of carbohydrates has rebounded to 500 g/d, but without a proportional increase in dietary fiber. This reflects a general increase in consumption of refined carbohydrates over the past 40–50 years (Gross, Li et al. 2004). Carbohydrate intake as a proportion of energy increased by 23% in men and almost 40% in women between 1977 and 2000 (Hite, Feinman et al. 2010).

This change in carbohydrate is consistent with the Dietary Guidelines for Americans, which was introduced in 1977 by the United States Department of Agriculture (USDA). This document recommended that Americans increase their intake of carbohydrate in place of total fat, saturated fat, cholesterol, and salt to reduce the risk of cardiovascular disease. These recommendations have persisted, and are generally reflected in today's guidelines. In 2002, the Institute of Medicine (IOM) set an acceptable macronutrient distribution range (AMDR) for carbohydrates of 45% to 65% of total energy intake, with a

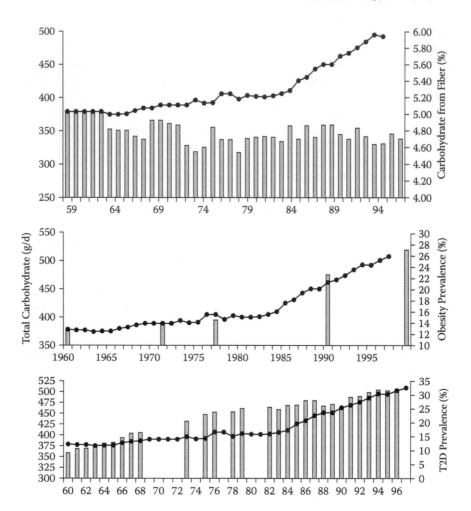

Figure 2.2 Carbohydrate intake and prevalence of obesity and T2D in US adults from 1960 to 1996. (Adapted from Gross, Li et al. 2004. *Am J Clin Nutr* **79**(5): 774–779.)

recommended maximal intake level of 25% or less of total calories from added sugar (Food and Nutrition Board (2002/2005); Dietary Reference Intakes for Energy).

Most of the increase in carbohydrate intake in the United States is due to refined grains, potatoes, and sugars—much of which are present as processed foods. These include sweetened grain products and desserts, pizza, potato/corn chips, rice, bread, beer, french fries/frozen potatoes, and sugar-sweetened beverages (SSBs) (Willett 2001). SSBs in fact provide one of the largest sources of calories to the US diet (Johnson, Appel et al. 2009). Between the late 1970s and 2006, the per capita consumption of SSB increased twofold from 64.4 kcal/d to 141.7 kcal/d, with adolescent and young adults consuming over 200 kcal/d (Popkin 2010). In 2004, SSBs contributed nearly 8% of total energy intake (Duffey and Popkin 2008), which exceed the American Heart Association's (2009) recommended upper limit of 100 kcal/d for most women and 150 kcal/d for most men from added sugars (Johnson, Appel et al. 2009).

In the United States, increases in carbohydrate intake correlate with increases in overweight (Body Mass Index [BMI] $\geq$ 25 kg/m²), obesity (BMI $\geq$ 30 kg/m²), and type 2 diabetes (Gross, Li et al. 2004). The Organization of Economic Co-operation and Development (OECD) projects that unless trends change, 75% of people living in the United States will be overweight by 2020 (Willett, Howe et al. 1997). By this time, type 2 diabetes is projected to reach a prevalence of nearly 20% (Boyle, Thompson et al. 2010). However, this pattern is the opposite in developing countries. In China and India, traditional high-carbohydrate diets are being replaced with Western diets rich in processed foods and animal fat. At the same time, the prevalence of overweight and obesity is rapidly increasing. For example, between 1991 and 1997, total carbohydrate as a proportion of energy in China decreased from 69% to 60%, whereas total fat increased form 19% to 27% (Du, Lu et al. 2002). This accompanied an increase in overweight prevalence from 10% to 15% (Du, Lu et al. 2002).

Other nutrients and total energy intake should be considered as potential confounders of the relationship between carbohydrate intake, overweight, and type 2 diabetes. Since 1977, total energy intake in the United States has increased by 7% in men and 22% in women (Hite, Feinman et al. 2010). This trend, accompanied by persistently low levels of physical activity, suggests that recent energy imbalance plays a critical role in the rapid increases in prevalence of overweight, obesity, and type 2 diabetes (Hite, Feinman et al. 2010).

Total carbohydrate

Excess fat mass and weight gain, outside of normal growth in the first two decades of life, leads to insulin resistance and an increased risk of type 2 diabetes. Conversely, a decrease in carbohydrate intake without changes in fat and protein will lead to decreased fat mass, insulin resistance, and type 2 diabetes risk. This pathway is well defined epidemiologically—overweight and obesity are the strongest and most prevalent risk factors for type 2 diabetes. But while this pathway is important given the overall increased intake of energy from carbohydrate in the United States (Hite, Feinman et al. 2010), it is not specific to carbohydrate. Unbalanced increases in the intake of fat or protein can also disturb energy balance, leading to excess adipose tissue and weight gain.

Carbohydrate may also influence the risk of type 2 diabetes independent of total energy intake. One possible mechanism is through prolonged hyperglycemia and hyperinsulinemia in response to a high carbohydrate diet. This may lead to beta cell damage, and impair insulin secretion. Frequent insulinemia may also desensitize adipose and muscle tissue to insulin, promoting insulin resistance (Miller 1994). Other possible mechanisms include oxidative stress and inflammation, recognized as key components of the pathophysiology of type 2 diabetes (Spranger, Kroke et al. 2003; Hotamisligil 2006).

Overweight and obesity

Over the last 30 years, there has been a great deal of interest in the relationship between carbohydrate intake and body fat. Much of this is due to a best-selling book by Robert Atkins, which was published in 1972 (Atkins 2002). Atkins recommended a radical reduction in carbohydrate intake while allowing for ad libitum intake of protein and fat, at least initially. This was to force the body into utilizing other sources of energy such as fat, leading to mild ketosis and weight loss. These and other claims attributed to low-carbohydrate diets have recently encouraged a "low-carb" craze, which has also renewed an interest in Paleolithic diets (Konner and Eaton 2011).

At first glance, such advice seems suspect because a simple replacement of carbohydrate by other nutrients will not lead to any changes in weight if total energy stays the same. However, if one of the nutrients that replaces carbohydrate increases metabolic rate or satiety, most likely the case for protein, energy balance could be disturbed which would lead to weight loss.

One of the claims about low-carbohydrate diets is that they are more satisfying than traditional moderate- and high-carbohydrate diets. This may well be the case if low-carbohydrate diets are high in protein. In a recent systematic review of 14 short-term (2 minutes to 1 day duration) trials using high- and low-protein intake, 11 reported that a high-protein preload significantly increased participant perceptions of satiety (Halton and Hu 2004). The review also identified 8 out of 15 trials, which showed that energy intake following a high protein preload significantly decreased (Halton and Hu 2004). These findings suggest that low-carbohydrate diets enriched in protein may curb hunger and prevent overeating at subsequent meals. Unfortunately, the mechanism behind these findings is unknown. Blood amino acid concentrations are likely involved, which may act as part of a negative feedback loop on appetite regulatory centers in the brain. Another potentially important feature of protein is its thermic effect, which is defined as an increase in metabolic rate required for digestion, absorption, and elimination of nutrients. Compared to carbohydrate and fat, protein has a relatively high thermic effect, which is on average 27% of energy compared to 10% for carbohydrate and fat. (Westerterp, Wilson et al. 1999) Thus, low-carbohydrate diets enriched in protein may also be more energetically expensive, potentially resulting in weight loss or weight maintenance over extended periods of time.

In the last 10 years, ad libitum low-carbohydrate diets have been tested in randomized trials for their weight loss potential against traditional hypocaloric moderate and high-carbohydrate diets. In meta-analyses of randomized trials by Hession et al. (9 studies, combined $n = 345$) (Hession, Rolland et al. 2009) and Nordmann et al. (5 studies, combined $n = 447$) (Nordmann, Nordmann et al. 2006), participants randomized to low-carbohydrate diets lost significantly more weight than comparison diets inside of 6 months. However, in the review by Hession et al. (Hession, Rolland et al. 2009), which included more studies, there was no significant difference in weight loss between diets after 1 year, which appeared to be due to poor adherence on all diets [Figure 2.3]. In a recent randomized weight-loss trial ($n = 811$) comparing hypocaloric low (35% energy), moderate (45% energy), and high (65% energy) carbohydrate diets over 2 years, there was no significant difference in weight loss between any of the diets. As with other studies, adherence to the diets and attendance at clinic visits were the most significant predictors of weight loss (Sacks, Bray et al. 2009). These results suggest that ad libitum low-carbohydrate such as Atkins may be useful for short-term weight loss, but that this effect is strongly tied to adherence. This is a remarkable conclusion given that ad libitum low-carbohydrate diets are not specifically designed to be hypocaloric. Participants on these diets appear to limit energy intake subconsciously, which, combined with the higher metabolic cost of consuming protein, may be driving weight loss.

But while weight loss is achievable using any diet, it is extremely difficult to maintain. There are few data to suggest that low-carbohydrate diets are any different in this regard. Controlled trials providing participants with a high degree of counseling and assistance were relatively unsuccessful at maintaining adherence and weight loss longer than 1 or 2 years. This problem obviously becomes much greater if adherence is to be maintained over decades. However, if low-carbohydrate diets are introduced at an early age, or become culturally ingrained, it might be possible to increase adherence. Long-term observational studies of low-carbohydrate diets and weight gain have the potential to shed light on this subject, but they may be difficult to interpret because weight gain is known to alter reporting of dietary intake. For example, people who are obese tend to underreport their intake of total energy (Voss, Kroke et al. 1998) and sugar (Bingham, Luben et al. 2007).

Despite potential benefits, there are some concerns that following a low-carbohydrate diet for long periods of time could lead to health

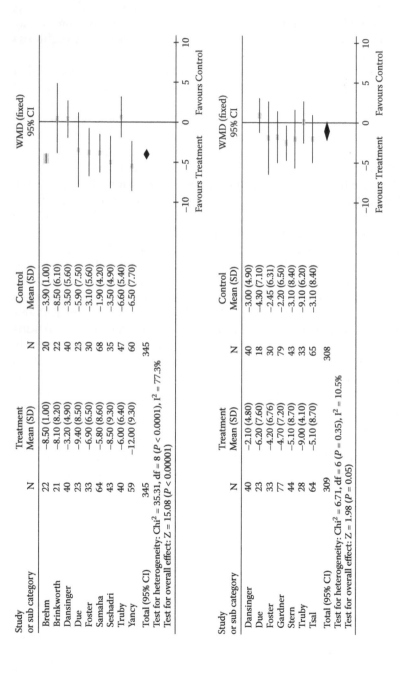

Figure 2.3 Meta-analysis of randomized trials of low-carbohydrate versus low-fat/calorie diets on short-term (top panel) and long-term (bottom panel) weight loss. (Adapted from Hession, Rolland et al. 2009.)

problems. For example, replacing carbohydrate with animal proteins and fat could lead to atherogenic lipid profiles and an increased risk of cardiovascular disease (Mensink, Zock et al. 2003). In the Nurses' Health Study (n = 82,802, cases = 1994, mean follow-up = 20 years) and Health Professionals Follow-up Study (n = 41,707, cases = 3289, mean follow-up = 20 years), participants adhering to low-carbohydrate diets were at an increased risk of suffering a fatal or non-fatal myocardial infarction if fat and protein were predominantly from animal sources (Halton, Willett et al. 2006; de Koning 2011). These findings are supported by a meta-analysis of 60 small trials showing an increase in LDL, although they did also raise HDL, for a replacement of carbohydrate with mainly animal-derived saturated fats (ΔLDL = 0.032 mmol/L, p < 0.001, ΔHDL = 0.010 mmol/L, p < 0.001). Also, in the Nurses' Health Study and Health Professionals' Follow-up Study, low-carbohydrate diets that replaced carbohydrate with vegetable protein and fat were associated with lower CHD risk (Halton, Willett et al. 2006; de Koning 2011). This too was supported by the same meta-analysis, showing that replacements of carbohydrates with monounsaturated fat (ΔHDL = 0.008 mmol/L, p < 0.001; ΔTriglycerides = −0.019 mmol/L, p < 0.001) or polyunsaturated fat (ΔHDL = 0.006 mmol/L, p < 0.001; ΔTriglycerides = −0.026 mmol/L, p < 0.001) raised HDL and lowered triglycerides.

Another worry about low-carbohydrate diets is that a correspondingly high protein intake has been associated with poor kidney function (Brenner, Lawler et al. 1996) and kidney stones (Curhan, Willett et al. 1993). However, in general, these associations are confined to those with preexisting kidney disease, and other studies disagree as to whether protein intake is truly a risk factor for kidney stones (Hiatt, Ettinger et al. 1996).

Type 2 diabetes

In order to assess whether carbohydrate is truly an independent factor in the etiology of type 2 diabetes risk, its effects must be isolated from total energy intake. As mentioned earlier, a change in energy intake can lead to a change in fat mass, which in itself is a predictor of type 2 diabetes risk. Also, if total energy intake is a diabetes risk factor independent of weight change, carbohydrate may appear to be related to type 2 diabetes risk simply because of higher energy intake. This means that for any assessment of carbohydrate etiology to be unbiased, energy intake and fat mass need to be held constant, either through statistical adjustments or through experimentation. However, even after controlling for energy, an association between carbohydrate and type 2 diabetes could still be due to a reciprocal change in protein, fat, or both. Thus, several other nutrients should be held constant, or different replacements tested, in order to pin down the effects of carbohydrate.

In an observational study, the estimated effect of carbohydrate is routinely isolated by controlling for energy and possible nutrient confounders in a regression model (Willett, Howe et al. 1997). This can be done by treating total carbohydrate as a covariate, or including residuals from separate regressions of total energy on carbohydrate intake. Controlling for total energy reduces confounding by total energy intake, as well as some confounding due to differences in body size, physical activity, and metabolic efficiency, which may be related to type 2 diabetes or lead to changes in energy intake (e.g., large individuals who consume more food will also consume more carbohydrate) (Willett, Howe et al. 1997). Controlling for energy intake also helps to cancel out correlated errors in the measurement of energy and carbohydrate intake by food frequency questionnaires (FFQs) (Willett, Howe et al. 1997). Statistical adjustment also allows several different nutrient substitutions to be simulated. For example, a substitution of carbohydrate for fat can be modeled by including terms for carbohydrate, protein, and energy in the same regression model. As all sources of energy are held constant except for fat, the interpretation of the term for carbohydrate is simply "changes in carbohydrate intake substituted for fat." A substitution of carbohydrate for protein is similarly modeled by including carbohydrate, fat, and total energy in the model.

There are numerous prospective observational studies of total carbohydrate intake and type 2 diabetes. In these studies, total carbohydrate intake has been inconsistently associated with type 2 diabetes risk. In the European Prospective Investigation into Cancer and Nutrition in the Netherlands (EPIC-NL, $n = 37,846$, cases = 915, mean follow-up = 10 years), one standard deviation increase in total carbohydrate intake was significantly associated with a 20% increase in the risk of developing type 2 diabetes (RR = 1.20, 95% CI: 1.01–1.42). Interestingly, this was independent of changes in the intake of other macronutrients (Sluijs, van der Schouw et al. 2011). Similar results were observed for starch and sugar; however, fiber was inversely associated with type 2 diabetes risk (RR = 0.89, 95% CI: 0.82–0.98) in this study (Sluijs, van der Schouw et al. 2011). Interestingly, in an analysis of a German sub-cohort from the same study (EPIC-Potsdam, $n = 25,067$, cases = 844, mean follow-up~10 years), total carbohydrate was inversely associated with type 2 diabetes risk provided it replaced protein (5% energy substitution, RR = 0.77, 95% CI: 0.64–0.91) or polyunsaturated fat (5% energy substitution, RR = 0.83, 95% CI: 0.70–0.98) (Schulze, Schulz et al. 2008). These results are at odds with the majority of other long-term prospective studies such as the Iowa Women's Health Study ($n = 35,988$, cases = 1141, mean follow-up = 6 years) (Meyer, Kushi et al. 2000), Nurses' Health Study ($n = 65,173$, cases = 915, mean follow-up = 6 years) (Salmeron, Manson et al. 1997), and the Health Professionals Follow-up Study ($n = 42,579$, cases = 523, mean follow-up = 6 years) (Salmeron, Ascherio et al. 1997), which did not found any significant association between total

carbohydrate intake and type 2 diabetes risk. All these studies comprehensively evaluated substitutions of carbohydrate for protein or total fat,
or adjusted for these nutrients.

Low-carbohydrate dietary patterns and their relationships with type
2 diabetes risk have also been investigated in both the Nurses' Health
Study (Halton, Liu et al. 2008) (n = 85,059, cases = 4670, follow-up = 20
years) and Health Professionals Follow-up Study (n = 40,475, cases = 2689,
follow-up = 20 years) (de Koning, Fung et al. 2011). Both studies utilized
scores that ranked participants according to their simultaneous intake of
carbohydrate, protein, and fat. Those consuming the highest percentage
of protein and fat but the lowest percentage of carbohydrate received the
highest score, whereas those consuming the lowest percentage of protein
and fat received the highest score. In these studies, participants consuming low-carbohydrate dietary patterns were at an increased risk of type
2 diabetes if total carbohydrate was replaced with animal fat, but were
at decreased risk if carbohydrate was replaced with vegetable fat. These
studies suggest that total carbohydrate is not as important to diabetes risk
compared to what it replaces in the diet. Unsaturated liquid vegetable fats
are thought to positively affect cell membrane fluidity, glucose transporter
function, and inflammation, and thus replacement of carbohydrate with
these components may result in some benefit (Riserus, Willett et al. 2009).

There have been several trials of total carbohydrate and type 2 diabetes risk; however, most have not examined incident type 2 diabetes as
the outcome. The main reason for this is that long-term dietary trials with
hard outcomes are technically challenging, and require long follow-up
periods to accrue a sufficient number of incident cases. Also, participants
in primary prevention studies are not as motivated to follow a dietary
intervention as those in secondary prevention studies, who have already
been diagnosed with type 2 diabetes. This often results in poor adherence
to the dietary interventions, and high dropout rates. As a consequence,
most trials are short-term and focus on changes in biomarkers among
those who already have type 2 diabetes or are overweight. Many are
also weight loss trials, which makes interpretation difficult as changes in
biomarker levels could be related to changes in fat mass or carbohydrate
intake. However, if the diet interventions in these studies produce equivalent weight change, or if weight change was controlled for in these studies, then carbohydrate–biomarker associations can be interpreted with a
minimum of bias. It should be noted, however, that even in the face of
equivalent weight change, a change in biomarkers could result from an
interaction between weight change and carbohydrate, or to differences in
body composition as discussed below.

In a trial, energy content of diets is fixed by designing diets that
exactly match changes in energy from carbohydrate with protein and

fat. Thus, dietary interventions will contain the same total energy, but different proportions of it will come from carbohydrate, fat, and protein.

For example, in the "Pounds Lost" trial, 811 initially overweight participants were randomized to four different diets—each with different carbohydrate contents of 35% E, 45% E, 55% E, and 65% E (Sacks, Bray et al. 2009). The respective fat and protein contributions for this study were 40% E/25% E, 40% E/15% E, 20% E/25% E, and 20% E/15% E (Sacks, Bray et al. 2009). While this study was designed as a weight-loss trial, with each diet being hypocaloric (750 kcal energy deficit), participants experienced identical weight loss, which means that changes in biomarkers are not confounded by changes in body fat. One important finding from this elegant study was that participants consuming the lowest-carbohydrate diet (35% E) had the greatest increase in HDL (+9% versus +6%, $p = 0.02$) compared to those consuming the highest-carbohydrate diet (65% E). And while serum insulin decreased significantly among all diet groups (6%–12%), it did not for the high-carbohydrate diet (Sacks, Bray et al. 2009). This suggests that low-carbohydrate diets may help to mitigate the most serious complication of type 2 diabetes—cardiovascular disease—and may be useful in improving glycemic control over the long term in people who are overweight. One possible explanation for this finding is a decrease in visceral fat. In a small weight-loss trial of 22 obese subjects with type 2 diabetics, those randomized to a low-carbohydrate diet (40% E) lost significantly more visceral fat over 4 weeks than subjects randomized to a high-carbohydrate diet (65% E)—despite there being no overall change in weight. Interestingly, this change accompanied a significant decrease in fasting insulin and an increase in HDL in the low-carbohydrate group (Miyashita, Koide et al. 2004).

However, not all trials of low-carbohydrate diets agree—especially regarding markers of glycemic control. In a 1 year parallel-group randomized trial of a low-carbohydrate "Atkins-style" (initial 20–25 g/day carbohydrate) diet versus a standard low-fat diet among 105 overweight adults with type 2 diabetes, participants experienced similar weight loss as well as decreases in glycosylated hemoglobin (HbA1c) (Davis, Tomuta et al. 2009). This was also observed in a 4-week parallel-arm weight loss trial of 47 overweight hyperlipidemic subjects, which compared a primarily vegetable-based Atkins-style low-carbohydrate (26% E) diet composed mostly of nuts, soy, fruits, vegetables, and cereals versus a high-carbohydrate lacto-ovo vegetarian diet (58% E) (Jenkins, Wong et al. 2009). In this study, participants lost similar weight (4.0 kg), but those randomized to the low-carbohydrate diet experienced a significantly greater decrease in LDL cholesterol. Glucose, insulin, and HbA1c all decreased significantly with both diets; however, there was no difference between them (Jenkins, Wong et al. 2009). Also, in a 4-week randomized crossover trial of 18 type 2 diabetic subjects, a high-carbohydrate (52% E) high-fiber

(28 g/1000 kcal) diet significantly lowered postprandial glucose, insulin, and triglycerides compared to a low-carbohydrate (45% E) high monounsaturated fat (23% E) diet (De Natale, Annuzzi et al. 2009). Other trials have found no evidence for low-carbohydrate diets superiority on modifying lipids in type 2 diabetics. For example, in 1 year randomized controlled trial of a low-carbohydrate high monounsaturated fat diet (45%%E, 20% E MUFA) versus a high carbohydrate low-fat diet (60%E, 25% E total fat) among 124 overweight subjects with type 2 diabetes, weight loss, HDL, LDL, and markers of glycemic control were not significantly different (Brehm, Lattin et al. 2009). And in a study of 320 Indians, an ethnic group uniquely predisposed to developing insulin resistance, while those randomized to a high-carbohydrate diet (> 70% E, mostly white rice) had significantly higher fasting glucose and insulin over 5 years compared to a reduced carbohydrate diet (<70% E), they had significantly lower triglycerides and very low density lipoprotein (VLDL) cholesterol (Mukherjee, Thakur et al. 2009).

The need for more specific and health-oriented classifications of carbohydrate

Together, these findings illustrate the heterogeneity of studies of carbohydrate intake, type 2 diabetes, and metabolic outcomes related to type 2 diabetes. Methodologic considerations such as the proportion of high-risk participants, weight change, energy intake, change in other nutrients, control for other dietary factors, and follow-up time make it extremely difficult to make an overall statement on the effect of total carbohydrate on type 2 diabetes and related biomarkers. But perhaps the greatest problem is that carbohydrate, similar to the other macronutrients, is heterogeneous.

Total carbohydrate is the sum of all forms of carbohydrates in the diet, such as processed foods including refined starch, refined sugar, and fiber isolates, but also whole foods such as grains, tubers, fruit, and vegetables. As it is now widely known that individual carbohydrates and even the foods they are found in have differing health effects, the net impact of total carbohydrate on type 2 diabetes risk will depend on their balance—as well as other components present in the diet. Thus, confounding is highly likely unless careful experiments and analyses are conducted, and carbohydrates that may have important favorable effects on health are separated from those that may not. Thus, simply enumerating total carbohydrate is not a valid approach to estimating risk.

The first recommendations regarding the health effects of carbohydrates centered on the avoidance of sugars such as sucrose, which are absorbed quickly by the body and lead to rapid increases in blood glucose and insulin. This characteristic hyperglycemia was used to justify replacements of dietary sugars with presumably more slowly digested complex carbohydrates including starches (Malik and Hu 2007). The rationale is that prolonged intake of sugar, and the corresponding prolonged elevations of glucose and insulin, may increase the risk of type 2 diabetes. Interestingly, few studies have actually demonstrated that intakes of dietary sugars are harmful for type 2 diabetes. For example, in a small trial where a 50 g serving of sucrose was given as a slice of cake as part of a high monounsaturated fat (20% E) diet for 24 days, no significant changes in glucose or insulin sensitivity were observed (Brynes and Frost 2007). In a small study of 12 type 2 diabetics, there were no overall changes in glycemia and insulinemia for isocaloric diets composed of 19% sucrose versus 3% sucrose with the same carbohydrate content (55% E) (Bantle, Swanson et al. 1993). Among observational studies, in a secondary analysis of the Women's Health Study (n = 39,435, cases = 918, mean follow-up = 6 years)—a randomized trial of aspirin and vitamin E for cardiovascular disease and cancer prevention— intakes of sucrose (top versus bottom quintile: RR = 0.84, 95% CI: 0.67– 1.04), fructose (RR = 0.96, 95% CI: 0.78–1.19), glucose (RR = 1.04, 0.85–1.28), and lactose (RR = 0.99, 0.80–1.22) were not significantly associated with type 2 diabetes risk (Janket, Manson et al. 2003). Similar findings were obtained in the Iowa Women's Health Study (n = 35,988, cases = 1141, mean follow-up = 6 years) for sucrose, which was not associated with increased risk; however, both glucose and fructose were positively associated with type 2 diabetes (Meyer, Kushi et al. 2000). Furthermore, it is now widely accepted that some complex carbohydrates are not digested more slowly than sugars. For example, starch from baked potatoes and white bread yield even greater glycemic responses than simple carbohydrates (Ludwig 2002). These findings have stimulated a reexamination of the health effects of carbohydrate, and the development of more nuanced health-related systems of classification.

Over the last 20–30 years, the concept of carbohydrate "quality" has evolved to represent the health-promoting aspects of carbohydrate, and embraces several partially overlapping but physiologically independent indicators. These include the glycemic index, glycemic load, amount and type of fiber, whole-grain integrity, degree of refinement, liquid verses solid sugar, and the newly developed insulin index and load. The information from these metrics is beginning to be incorporated into dietary recommendations. For example, in the most recent dietary recommendations for Americans, at least half of all grain products are recommended to be whole, added sugars are to be minimized, and sugar-sweetened beverages are to be replaced with noncaloric beverages such as water (United States Department of Agriculture 2010).

Glycemic index and glycemic load

The glycemic index (GI) was developed in 1981 by David Jenkins and colleagues at the University of Toronto in order to improve the management of type 1 diabetes. In recognition of its importance in promoting health, the World Health Organization recommended in 1998 that food manufacturers attempt to reduce the GI of prepared foods (World Health Organization/Food and Agriculture Organization 1998). GI is simply a ranking system that classifies foods according to postprandial glucose response following their consumption (Jenkins, Wolever et al. 1981). The index is scored from 0 to 100, and is a standardized comparison of blood glucose increase (2-h incremental area under the glucose response curve) following the ingestion of 50 g of carbohydrate from a test food versus an equivalent amount from a reference carbohydrate. This can be either glucose or white bread, both of which are assigned a GI of 100. Foods with a GI greater than 70 are arbitrarily considered "high GI," while those with a GI less than 55 are considered "low GI" (Atkinson, Foster-Powell et al. 2008) [Table 2.1]. High GI foods that are commonly consumed in the US diet include SSBs (e.g., cola = 90) and hard candy (GI = 99). Common low GI foods include most whole fruits and vegetables (e.g., apples, GI = 38) (Atkinson, Foster-Powell et al. 2008). The GI of a complex meal is calculated

Table 2.1 Examples of Glycemic Index and Glycemic Load Values of Some Common Foods

Food	Serving size (g)	Carbohydrate (g)	Glycemic index	Glycemic load
White bread	30	14	70	10
Whole-wheat bread	30	11	68	7
Pancakes, homemade	80	26	66	17
Bran flakes	30	18	74	13
Oatmeal, cooked	250	21	42	9
Muffin, bran	57	24	60	14
Doughnut, cake	47	23	76	17
Apple, raw	120	16	40	6
Banana, raw	120	24	47	11
Lentils, green–boiled	150	14	37	5
Beans, navy–boiled	150	30	31	9
Carrots, diced and boiled	80	5	49	2
Potato, white–boiled	150	26	96	24
Cola soft drink	250	26	63	16
Orange juice, from concentrate	250	26	57	15

by multiplying the GI of each individual food by its carbohydrate content, and dividing by the total carbohydrates consumed in the meal.

The GI of a food depends on its rate of digestion and absorption, which is influenced by many factors. For example, starch gelatinization refers to the extent that starch particles swell in water, which has a significant effect on GI. A higher water content allows starch to react much more quickly with amylases, which hydrolyze the starch polymers into glucose. Boiled and baked potatoes are good examples of foods with very high starch gelatinization, which gives them a higher GI than the poorly gelatinized starch of some brown rices. Particle size is also an important consideration. Small, finely ground starch granules found in cornstarch and white flour have a very high surface area which increases the number of available sites that amylases can act on, thereby raising GI (Hu 2010). Many common pastries comprised of predominantly white wheat flour have a GI of over 100, which is higher than that of table sugar (Atkinson, Foster-Powell et al. 2008). Refinement also strips grains of bran, which is the major source of fiber and may impact GI. For example, soluble fiber present in pulses (e.g., lentils) and some cereals (e.g., oats and barley) slows the digestion of starches by forming an undigestible gel that lowers GI. Insoluble fiber, which is mostly found in cereals and vegetables, increases gastric motility and may limit digestion. This is one of the reasons why some, but not all, whole grains have a lower GI than refined grains. Another important factor in determination of GI is the ratio of amylose to amylopectin. Grains with a higher percentage of amylose instead of amylopectin have lower glycemic responses because amylose is more resistant to digestion than amylopectin (Behall, Scholfield et al. 1988). GI is also affected by pH (↓ pH, ↓ GI), cooking time and method (↑ cooking, ↑ GI), ripeness (↑ GI), fat and protein content (↓ GI), and simple grain integrity (↓ GI) (Harris and Kris-Etherton 2010; Thorne, Thompson et al. 1983).

To reflect a measure of both carbohydrate quality and quantity, the glycemic load (GL) was developed by Walter Willett and colleagues at the Harvard School of Public Health (Salmeron, Manson et al. 1997). GL is defined as the product of GI and carbohydrate content for a given food, and is calculated for a meal by simply adding together the GI * carbohydrate products for each food. The GL helps to resolve some of the measurement issues associated with the GI—especially those with fruits and vegetables. For example, a serving of boiled, diced carrots has a GI of 49—which is the same as a serving of boiled spaghetti (Atkinson, Foster-Powell et al. 2008). While the GI for carrots reflects the high per unit potency of its sugars, it is an unrealistically high number because the amount of available carbohydrate in carrots is extremely small (5 g/serving) compared to spaghetti (48 g/serving). After multiplying these figures together, the GL for a serving of carrots is 2, whereas for spaghetti it is 24 (Atkinson, Foster-Powell et al. 2008). One special point about the GL is that it is correlated with total carbohydrate because total carbohydrate is included in its calculation. This has some implications for the interpretation of data from carbohydrate analyses. Changes in risk that are associated with GL are partially, perhaps mostly, due to carbohydrate content and vice versa.

Large international projects are currently underway to create comprehensive databases of GI values (e.g., http://www.glycemicindex.com/). However, these efforts are complicated by the obvious requirement that GI must be derived experimentally. This is a time consuming and costly process that is not coordinated by a central laboratory. Rather, GI values are collected from diverse sources such as food industry data, academic research laboratories, and graduate student theses. This makes it very difficult to ensure consistency in testing methodology, which can increase variation in GI values for the same food. Differences in processing, cooking methods, ripeness, can further increase GI variation—which makes GI a fundamentally error-prone measure, not unlike the measure of most dietary components, which are also based on a variety of assumptions. Further, if a food of interest is not present in a GI database, a researcher may have to impute values from similar foods. This may not be a valid approach; however, in the absence of experimentally derived data, it may be the only solution.

Overweight and obesity

The heightened interest in low-carbohydrate diets has extended to include concepts of GI and GL which, despite inconsistencies in the data, have been incorporated into popular weight loss regimes. In fact, many low-carbohydrate diets are also low GI or GL because they replace carbohydrate-rich foods with fat and protein-rich foods. However, this is not the only way to produce a low GI/GL diet. A low GI/GL diet can be constructed by exchanging high GI/GL foods such as cooked potatoes, white bread, and refined breakfast cereals with low GI/GL carbohydrate foods including lentils, whole grain bread, and cooked breakfast cereals (Pereira, Swain et al. 2004). This way, total carbohydrate can be maintained in the moderate range (e.g., 45% E–60% E).

As with low-carbohydrate diets, low GI or GL diets may enhance weight loss by reducing hunger or improving satiety. However, one of the specific mechanisms by which low GI/GL diets are hypothesized to promote weight loss is by lowering postprandial insulin, and maintaining high insulin sensitivity (Abete, Astrup et al. 2010). This may lead to a reduced hunger response and minimize overeating (Esfahani, Wong et al. 2009).

Several controlled trials have examined the role of GI and GL in weight loss. In a 2007 Cochrane review and meta-analysis of six small randomized weight loss trials (combined n = 202, follow-up = 5 weeks–6 months), low GI or GL diets promoted on average a significant weight loss of 1 kg, fat mass loss of 1 kg, and a BMI reduction of 1.3 kg/m^2 compared to either high GI/GL or low-fat diets (Thomas, Elliott et al. 2007). Most of the diets used in these studies did not rely on foods high in protein and fat (e.g., meat, dairy) to lower GI and GL. Rather, they focused on whole-grain versions of carbohydrate-rich foods that participants usually ate, for example, whole-grain bread, brown rice, cooked breakfast cereals, and lentils. These were consumed along with participants' usual selections of protein and fat-enriched foods (Slabber, Barnard et al. 1994; Bouche, Rizkalla et al. 2002; Ebbeling, Leidig et al. 2003; Sloth, Krog-Mikkelsen et al. 2004; Ebbeling, Leidig et al. 2005). Two studies did, however, include dairy in a list of foods recommended to participants in order to meet GI targets (Ebbeling, Leidig et al. 2003, 2005). Only one study promoted lean red meats and animal proteins to help lower GI—however, this diet was tested in combination with both low GI carbohydrates and high GI carbo-hydrates (McMillan-Price, Petocz et al. 2006). Interestingly, carbohydrate content in all these diets was maintained between 45%–65% E, which was significantly higher than in low-carbohydrate trials that focused exclusively on carbohydrate reduction. However, there were some major differences between the interventions—some were hypocaloric while others were ad libitum. The authors concluded that in studies compar-ing ad libitum low GI diets to energy restricted low GI diets, participants lost as much or more weight than the standard low GI diets. In a more recent (2008) and comprehensive meta-regression analysis that evaluated weight loss in low versus high GI/GL diets among 23 trials lasting more than 1 week, body weight significantly decreased following a reduction in dietary GL (Livesey, Taylor et al. 2008). This was optimized when GL was reduced by more than 17 units per day, but was most consistent when the difference was greater than 42 units per day. (Livesey, Taylor et al. 2008). The overall benefit was calculated as -1.7 g/week for a 1 GL unit decrease per day; however, this was confined to studies where conditions were ad libitum (Livesey, Taylor et al. 2008). These findings are similar to those from trials of ad libitum low-carbohydrate diets, which found that unrestricted intake of certain foods results in weight loss. This reinforces the point that calorie reduction may be less important than consuming satisfying foods. However, clearly longer and larger trials are needed to substantiate these results. Most studies were of very short duration, and the heterogeneity in participants and design suggest that results should be interpreted with caution.

As for observational studies, there have been very few prospective cohort studies of GI or GL on weight gain, and their findings have not been consistent. In a small study by Ma et al. (n = 572, mean follow-up = 1 year), GI but not GL or total carbohydrate was significantly associated with increased BMI (Ma, Olendzki et al. 2005). In a subsample of the Danish arm of the monitoring Trends and Determinants in cardiovascular disease study (n = 376, mean follow-up = 6 years), higher GI was associated with significantly higher body weight, body fat, and waist circumference in women but not in men (Hare-Bruun, Flint et al. 2006). GL was not associated with weight gain in this study (Hare-Bruun, Flint et al. 2006), and a number of potential limitations that may explain the inconsistency in the findings were described by Pereira (Pereira 2006). In a large study including participants from five European countries (n = 89,432, mean follow-up = 6.5 years), GI and GL were not significantly associated with weight change; however, high GI was associated with a larger waist circumference (Du, van der et al. 2009). However, in this study, associations were highly heterogeneous by center, which makes interpretation difficult.

Despite inconsistencies in the data, the insulinemia mechanism seems to be one of the best explanations for why low GI/GL diets may promote weight loss. In a recent randomized trail of a low GI versus low fat diet, an above-median 30-min insulin level following a 75 g glucose load modified the weight loss effect of a low GI/GL diet (Ebbeling, Leidig et al. 2007). Participants with a high insulin response lost significantly more weight and body fat on the low GI/GL versus a low-fat diet compared to those with a lower insulin response (Ebbeling, Leidig et al. 2007). Thus, participants who are insulin resistant or secrete more insulin may be more likely to benefit from a low GI/GL diet. A reduction in hyperinsulinemia may also promote weight loss because of its connection to de novo lipogenesis in animal models (Esfahani, Wong et al. 2009). Low GI/GL diets may also limit the release of gastrointestinal hormones that may also help to blunt insulin release and maintain satiety. In a 10-week trial of 29 overweight women, a low GI diet reduced plasma glucose-like peptide 1 (GLP-1) levels, which facilitates insulin secretion following ingestion of glucose; however, the glucose-dependent insulinotropic polypeptide GIP, which has a similar function, was not affected (Krog-Mikkelsen, Sloth et al. 2011).

Fiber content may also help to explain why low GI/GL diets promote satiety (Pereira and Ludwig 2001). For example, in a number of small feeding studies, low GI foods that were high in fiber such as oatmeal and legumes increased participant's perception of fullness better than low-fiber foods, which lead to decreased food intake at subsequent meals (Ludwig 2000). Conversely, high GI foods and SSBs increased subsequent hunger and decrease satiety (Roberts 2000). These and other studies indicate that high fiber low GI versus high GI foods may help to control overeating and maintain body weight (Roberts 2000).

However, despite the numerous lines of evidence suggesting a role for GI and GL in weight loss, the 2010 dietary guidelines for Americans concluded that GI and GL are not associated with body weight and do not lead to greater weight loss or better weight maintenance (United States Department of Agriculture 2010). The reason for this position is based on the heterogeneous nature of supporting data. For example, in a 2004 Cochrane meta-analysis evaluating trials of low GI diets and body weight (Kelly, Frost et al. 2004) and two qualitative reviews including more recent trials (Gaesser 2007; Vega-Lopez and Mayol-Kreiser 2009), GI and GL were not related to weight loss. And in the most recent long-term trials, only a small benefit of low GI/GL diets was seen before 8 weeks of follow-up, after which there was no benefit. This was observed in both ad libitum or either energy-restricted conditions. As with low-carbohydrate diets, this may be related to adherence. Therefore, larger and more carefully con-ducted studies of GI and GL are needed to resolve this question.

Type 2 diabetes

Early studies, which evaluated the impact of low GI/GL foods, consis-tently found that peak postprandial blood glucose and insulin were much lower following their consumption (Esfahani, Wong et al. 2009). This shift toward modest but prolonged postprandial glycemia and insulinemia is thought to reduce the risk of developing type 2 diabetes (Esfahani, Wong et al. 2009). Prolonged insulin secretion associated with low GI/GL diets is hypothesized to suppress serum free fatty acid concentrations, but also the counter-regulator response involving glucagon and other hormones that occur during significant swings in plasma glucose (Esfahani, Wong et al. 2009). Reduced free fatty acids helps to prevent lipid accumulation in muscle and liver cells, which disrupts insulin signaling and glycemic control, both of which are characteristics of insulin resistance (Samuel, Petersen et al. 2010). The repeated high and transient hyperinsulinemia associated with high GI/GL diets may elevate serum free fatty acid levels and down-regulate the expression of somatic insulin receptors, thereby initiating a self-perpetuating cycle of hyperinsulinemia and insulin resis-tance that stresses the beta cell (Ludwig 2002). In addition, high GI/GL diets may impair beta cell function directly through elevated glucose (glucotoxicity) and fatty acid (lipotoxicity) concentrations (Ludwig 2002). Over the last 25 years, numerous observational studies and clinical trials have sought to determine whether the effects of GI and GL are consistent with these mechanisms. And although findings have been mixed, larger studies generally indicate a moderate positive association between GI or GL and risk of developing type 2 diabetes, which is supported by findings from randomized trials examining markers of glycemic control.

Among prospective cohort studies, GI and GL have been associated with an increased risk of type 2 diabetes in several large and influen-tial studies such as the Nurses' Health Study (Salmeron, Manson et al. 1997) and Health Professionals Follow-up Study (Salmeron, Ascherio et al. 1997). However, in other independent cohort studies, these associations were not replicated. For example, in the Iowa Women's Health Study, both

GI and GL were not significantly associated with risk of type 2 diabetes despite this study having a large sample size (n = 35,988), relatively long follow-up (6 years), and large number of incident cases (n = 1141) (Meyer, Kushi et al. 2000). This was also observed in the Atherosclerosis Risk in Communities (ARIC) study, which contained 12,251 participants, 1,447 cases over 9 years of follow-up (Stevens, Ahn et al. 2002). These and other discrepant results have cast some doubt on whether GI and GL are etiologically linked to type 2 diabetes risk. However, these null findings may have been due to measurement error. If the assessment of GI or GL includes substantial random error, the true association between GI/GL and type 2 diabetes may be biased toward the null. This point was addressed in a 2008 meta-analysis of six prospective cohort studies by Barclay et al. (Barclay, Petocz et al. 2008) (Figure 2.4), which was notable in that it included only studies where the correlation of carbohydrate measured by FFQ to carbohydrate measured by diet records was greater than 0.5. This cutoff is generally regarded as the lower limit of a FFQ's ability to rank participants by nutrient intake (Brunner, Stallone et al. 2001). Incidentally, both the Iowa Women's Health Study and the ARIC study reported validation coefficients of 0.45 and so were excluded from the analysis. Several other studies were eliminated for not having established the validity of their FFQs in populations that were similar to the ones being studied, which could lead to a poor assessment of usual dietary GI and GL. After these exclusions, the results of the meta-analysis were clear. Both GI and GL were strong predictors of incident type 2 diabetes. In the meta-analysis, the top versus the bottom quintile of GI was associated with a 40% increase in risk (RR = 1.40, 95% CI: 1.23–1.59), whereas for GL, the same comparison was associated with a 27% increase in risk. (RR = 1.27, 95% CI: 1.12–1.45) (Barclay, Petocz et al. 2008). Other more recent prospective cohort studies that were not included in this analysis included three (Barclay, Flood et al. 2007; Krishnan, Rosenberg et al. 2007; Villegas, Liu et al. 2007) that reported significant positive associations with GI and type 2 diabetes either in primary or stratified analysis, and two (Mosdol, Witte et al. 2007; Sahyoun, Anderson et al. 2008) reporting no association. Among others evaluating GL, two reported positive associations (Villegas, Liu et al. 2007; Halton, Liu et al. 2008), two found no association (Krishnan, Rosenberg et al. 2007; Sahyoun, Anderson et al. 2008), and one study found an inverse association that was attenuated after adjusting for fiber and carbohydrate (Mosdol, Witte et al. 2007). In the recent large analysis of the EPIC-Netherlands study (n = 37,846, mean follow-up = 10 years), dietary GL was associated with an increased risk of diabetes (RR = 1.32 per 1 SD increase, 95% CI: 1.14–1.54), whereas GI was more weakly associated with diabetes risk (RR = 1.08, 95% CI: 1.0–1.17) (Sluijs, van der Schouw et al. 2010). Findings from the Nurses' Health Study also indicates that a high dietary GL increases the risk of cholesterol gallstone disease,

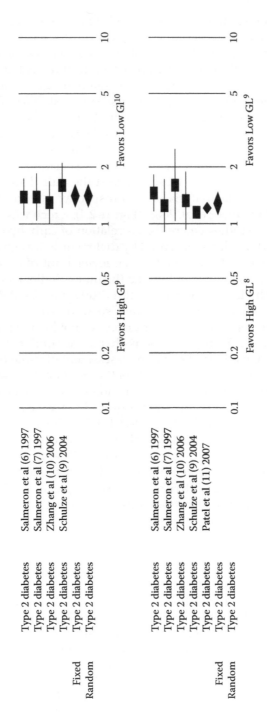

Figure 2.4 Meta-analysis of the relationship between glycemic index and load with T2D among prospective studies. (From Barclay, Petocz et al. 2008. *Am J Clin Nutr* **87**(3): 627–637.)

which is associated with insulin resistance, type 2 diabetes, and the metabolic syndrome (Tsai, Leitzmann et al. 2005).

Among randomized trials, a Cochrane review published in 2009 that included 11 randomized trials lasting 1 to 12 months among 402 participants with diabetes (3 trials in type 1 diabetes, 7 trials in type 2 diabetes, and 1 trial in both) indicated that low GI diets versus high GI or other diets reduced markers of glycemic control (Thomas and Elliott 2009). In this study, HbA1c levels were reduced by 0.5% (95% CI: −0.8 to −0.2, $p <$ 0.001) (Thomas and Elliott 2009), which is similar to reductions obtained using medication for patients with type 2 diabetes (Esfahani, Wong et al. 2009). Fructosamine (glycosylated serum proteins), which is a shorter-term marker of glycemic control than HbA1c, was reduced by 0.23% (95% CI: −0.47 to 0.00, $p =$ 0.05) and hypoglycemic episodes were significantly decreased with low GI diets compared to high GI diets. Similar findings have been reported in other meta-analyses, which also indicate a significant inverse association with fasting plasma glucose (Brand-Miller, Hayne et al. 2003; Livesey, Taylor et al. 2008; Sievenpiper, Kendall et al. 2009). These results were also seen in a 6-month trial comparing a low GI versus a high cereal fiber diet among 210 patients with type 2 diabetes who were also using oral antidiabetic agents (Jenkins, Kendall et al. 2008); however, a larger and longer trial managed by diet alone did not find an effect of a low GI diet on HbA1c (Wolever, Gibbs et al. 2008). This finding has been suggested to be due to low baseline levels (mean 6.1%) (Wolever, Gibbs et al. 2008). While several studies have reported improvements in fasting blood glucose in low GI/GL diets compared to other diets, inconsistent results have been observed for fasting insulin and insulin sensitivity, which may be due to insulin levels being less variable in normal weight individuals (Thomas, Elliott et al. 2007; Livesey, Taylor et al. 2008; Thomas and Elliott 2009).

GI and GL have also been associated with changes in inflammatory factors. For example, in the Canadian Trial of Carbohydrates in Diabetes (CCD), which tested three diets (high GI + high carb, low GI + low carb, low carb + high MUFA) over 1 year on changes in HbA1c and C-reactive protein (CRP), the low GI diet significantly reduced CRP levels by 30% compared to the high GI diet (Wolever, Gibbs et al. 2008). In a cross-sectional analysis of the Women's Health Study ($n =$ 244), CRP in the top quintile of glycemic load was 95% higher than in the bottom quintile after adjusting for potential confounders (Liu, Manson et al. 2002). Interestingly, this association was much stronger (+212%) among women who were overweight (BMI > 25 kg/m^2, p for interaction = 0.01) (Liu, Manson et al. 2002). In a much larger sample from the same study ($n =$ 18,137), a similar overall association was observed for GI but not GL (Levitan, Cook et al. 2008). Finally, in a cross-sectional sample of diabetic women from the Nurses' Health Study ($n =$ 902), dietary GI was significantly associated with increased levels of CRP and the tumor necrosis factor alpha receptor 2 (TNF-R2) (Qi, van Dam et al. 2006). While the mechanism behind these relationships is poorly understood, hyperglycemia is known to increase the production of superoxide radicals via the electron transport chain, which could initiate an inflammatory response (Brownlee 2001; Esposito, Nappo et al. 2002). Another possibility is that increased inflammation is simply a consequence of the intracellular dysfunction (e.g., ER stress) characteristic of insulin resistance and type 2 diabetes (Hotamisligil 2006). Increased levels of inflammatory factors might therefore simply represent disease severity, rather than a direct causal link with GI and GL. This could also be the case with adiponectin, a hormone secreted by adipose tissue that is associated with improvements in insulin sensitivity, inflammation, and glycemic control (Qi, Rimm et al. 2005; Montonen, Drogan et al. 2011). In cross-sectional studies of diabetic men from the Health Professionals Follow-up Study (Qi, Rimm et al. 2005) ($n = 780$) and diabetic women ($n = 902$) from the Nurses Health Study (Qi, Meigs et al. 2006), glycemic index and load were inversely associated with adiponectin concentrations.

Fiber

While fiber intake has been associated with a number of important health benefits, the average consumption of dietary fiber in US adults is approximately 15 g per day—which is far below the recommended intake of 14 g per 1000 kcal (~25 g per day for a 2000 kcal/day diet) (Slavin 2008). This pales in comparison to what is thought to be the fiber intake of some early Paleolithic diets, estimated at up to 100 g per day or more (Eaton 2006). The major sources of fiber in the US diet are white wheat flour, which provides 16% of all fiber consumed, and potatoes, which provide 9%. While these are not concentrated sources of fiber, they are widely consumed, which accounts for their disproportionate contributions. They are also very high GI/GL—which is generally not the case for high fiber foods. The most concentrated food sources of dietary fiber are whole grains, legumes, vegetables, nuts, and dried fruits—which are low GI/GL. However, in the US diet, these are not consumed frequently (Slavin 2008).

While dietary fiber is generally defined as the nondigestible carbohydrates found in plants, this definition has been recently expanded to include oligosaccharides such as inulin and resistant starches—which include both starch and starch-degradation products which bypass digestion in the small intestine to be fermented in the colon (Slavin 2008). Resistant starch is found in seeds, legumes, and unprocessed whole grains, but is also formed during cooking and cooling of starch-containing foods such as cooked-and-chilled potatoes and parboiled rice (Harris and

Kris-Etherton 2010). Current intake of resistant starch in the United States is estimated to be between 4 and 8 g per day, and 60% is provided from breads, cooked pasta, and vegetables (Murphy, Douglass et al. 2008).

The chief physiologic effect of dietary fiber is that it delays gastric emptying, which contributes to a feeling of "fullness" and prolonged satiety (Pereira and Ludwig 2001). However, soluble fiber, which dissolves in water to form a gel, is unique in that it traps and delays the absorption of nutrients. This tends to blunt postprandial glycemia, lipemia, and insulin responses (Howarth, Saltzman et al. 2001). Soluble fiber is also readily fermented by colonic bacteria to produce short-chain fatty acids (SCFA), which increase hepatic insulin sensitivity and decrease hepatic lipogenesis (Schulze, Schulz et al. 2007). This is arguably its most important physiologic function (Weickert and Pfeiffer 2008).

The main benefit obtained from insoluble fiber is an increase in fecal bulking and laxity. Insoluble fibers may also undergo some fermentation in the colon; however, this process is poorly understood. Soluble fiber, insoluble fiber, and resistant starch that escape digestion but provide a fermentation substrate for gut bacteria are termed *prebiotics*.

Overweight and obesity

Among prospective cohort studies, dietary fiber appears to be associated with weight maintenance and may be useful for preventing overweight and obesity (Ludwig, Pereira et al. 1999). In a meta-analysis of four prospective cohort studies (combined $n = 111,789$), participants who consumed the highest level of fiber had a 30% lower risk of developing obesity (BMI $\geq$ 30) compared to participants with the lowest level of fiber intake (RR = 0.70 95% CI = 0.62, 0.78) (Anderson, Baird et al. 2009). This was confirmed in a recent pooled analysis of data from 6 countries in the EPIC study (combined $n = 89,432$, mean follow-up = 6.5 years), where a 10 g per day increase in total fiber intake was associated with a 39 g decrease in body weight per year (95% C: −71 to −7). A similar relationship was also observed for waist circumference in this study (−0.08 cm per year, 95% CI: −0.11 to −0.05) (Du, van der et al. 2010). Interestingly, the relationship with body weight in this study was attributed to cereal fiber (−77 g/year, 95% CI: −127 to −26), whereas fruit and vegetable fiber were not significantly associated with weight change. Interestingly, fruit and vegetable fiber were inversely associated with waist circumference. In an analysis of fiber intake trends from the Nurses' Health Study ($n = $ 74,091) women who increased their cereal fiber intake the most (top quintile), over 12 years of follow-up gained on average 1.52 kg less than women who increased their cereal fiber intake the least (bottom quintile; p for trend <0.0001) (Liu, Willett et al. 2003). Similar findings were observed in the Health Professionals' Follow-up Study ($n = 27,082$), at least for cereal fiber. In this study, every 20 g per day increase in cereal fiber was associated with a 0.81 kg reduction in 8-year weight gain (Koh-Banerjee, Franz et al. 2004). However, this rose to 2.51 kg for fiber from fruit (p for trends < 0.0001) (Koh-Banerjee, Franz et al. 2004). And in a smaller sample from the same study (n = 16,587), a 12 g per day increase in total fiber was associated with a 0.63 cm decrease in waist circumference gain over 9 years of follow-up (p for trend < 0.0001) (Koh-Banerjee, Chu et al. 2003).

Among small trials, increased fiber intake helps to quell hunger, promote satiety, decrease voluntary energy intake, and maintain body weight (Howarth, Saltzman et al. 2001; Pereira and Ludwig 2001). In a small meta-analysis of 15 short-term trials, a fiber supplement (guar gum or glucomannan) added to a hypocaloric diet promoted significantly greater weight loss compared to the placebo-supplemented diet at 4 (–1.7 kg, 95% CI: –1.3 to –2.0) and 8 (–2.4 kg, 95% CI: –1.9 to –2.9) weeks, but not at 12 weeks— which may be because only 9 trials were included in the 12-week time point (Anderson, Baird et al. 2009). Among studies allowing for ad libitum energy intake, a 14 g per day increase in fiber resulted in 10% lower energy intake and a 1.9 kg weight loss over 3.8 months (Howarth, Saltzman et al. 2001). Interestingly, these effects were much stronger among obese versus non-obese participants (18 versus 6% lower energy intake, 2.4 versus 8 kg decreased body weight) (Howarth, Saltzman et al. 2001). However, an earlier meta-analysis of 34 small trials using guar gum supplement did not find any significant weight loss benefit (Pittler and Ernst 2001). As well, trials have failed to demonstrate any important difference between soluble and insoluble fiber in relation to weight control (Weickert and Pfeiffer 2008). This could be because of the relatively consistent association between fiber intake and body weight management in epidemiologic studies, which is due to the combined effects of components in foods rather than fiber itself. Fiber from foods could also have different effects than fiber from supplements (Hu 2008; Anderson, Baird et al. 2009). At the present time, there are no human studies specifically addressing resistant starch intake and weight change; however, in rodent models, resistant starch appears to prevent weight gain or regain during overfeeding with high-fat diets (Higgins, Jackman et al. 2010; Shimotoyodome, Suzuki et al. 2010).

Increased fiber intake may lead to decreased energy intake through a variety of mechanisms. For example, fiber (1) displaces energy in the diet, (2) increases chewing that limits food intake, (3) increases production of saliva and gastric juice that expands the stomach and increases satiety, (4) delays gastric emptying and intestinal absorption of nutrients (mostly soluble viscous fiber) that leads to reduced postprandial glucose and insulin (Slavin 2008) and hunger response (Hu 2008), (5) increases the secretion of satiety-related gut hormones (Weickert and Pfeiffer 2008), and (6) increases fecal energy loss via shorter intestinal transit time (Miller and Judd 1984). Resistant starch and some types of fiber may also alter gut microbiota, which could reduce caloric availability and perhaps induce weight loss over time (Harris and Kris-Etherton 2010).

Type 2 diabetes

In a 2008 position paper, the American Dietetic Association concluded that diets that provide 30 to 50 g of fiber per day from whole foods yield lower blood glucose compared to low-fiber diets (Slavin 2008). Most of this effect is attributed to soluble fiber, which slows the rate of digestion and absorption of glucose and should help to improve glycemic control and insulin sensitivity. This effect is illustrated in a meta-analysis of randomized trials testing the glycemic effect of adding small amounts of the low-viscosity soluble fiber maltodextrin to common carbohydrate-rich foods (e.g., white rice, bread, and sugar-sweetened beverages) (Livesey and Tagami 2009). On average, 6 g of maltodextrin per serving lowers the glycemic response by 10% in solid foods, but 20% in liquid foods (Livesey and Tagami 2009). However, among long-term epidemiologic studies of type 2 diabetes, mostly insoluble cereal fiber appears to be associated with greatest health benefits. In a meta-analysis of eight prospective cohort studies, intake of cereal fiber (mostly insoluble fiber from wheat, some soluble fiber from oats, barley, etc.) but not fruit (mostly soluble fiber) and vegetable fiber (mostly insoluble fiber) was associated with a lower risk of type 2 diabetes (top versus bottom category RR = 0.67, 95% CI: 0.62–0.72) (Schulze, Schulz et al. 2007). One possible explanation for this discrepancy is the very low intake of fruit and vegetables versus whole-grain cereals in the studies included (Venn and Mann 2004).

Interestingly, diets with the lowest GI/GL and highest fiber content appear to be associated with the lowest risk of type 2 diabetes, whereas diets with the highest GI/GL and the lowest fiber content are associated with the highest risk. At first glance, this seems obvious because many high-fiber foods are also low GI/GL. However, fiber is one of many determinants of GI/GL, and so there is still some residual variation in fiber that is not accounted for by GI/GL. In a meta-analysis by Livesey et al., the correlation between fiber and GL was as high as 0.88. However, this is likely an overestimate because of the aggregate nature of the data (Livesey, Taylor et al. 2008). In the Health Professionals Follow-up Study (n = 42,759, mean follow-up = 6 years, cases = 523), and the Nurses' Health Study (n = 65,173, mean follow-up = 6 years, cases = 915) [Figure 2.5], cereal fiber intake in the lowest quintile combined with a GL in the highest quintile was associated with at least a twofold higher risk of type 2 diabetes compared to a combination of the lowest quintiles (HPFS RR = 2.2 fold, 95% CI: 1.04–4.54; NHS RR = 2.5, 95% CI: 1.14–5.51; p for trend < 0.0001) (Salmeron, Ascherio et al. 1997; Salmeron, Manson et al. 1997). Similarly,

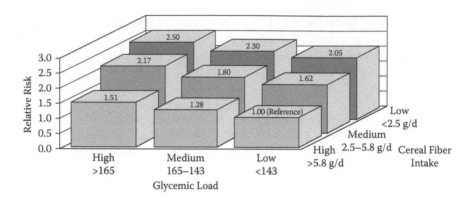

Figure 2.5 Cross-tabular relationship between glycemic load, cereal fiber intake, and T2D in the Nurses' Health Study. (From Salmeron, Manson et al. 1997.)

in a prospective cohort study of Hawaiian adults of various ethnicities (n = 75,512, mean follow-up = 14 years, cases = 8 587), participants in the top quintile of cereal fiber intake had a 10% lower risk of type 2 diabetes, and GL was positively associated with type 2 diabetes risk among Caucasians (Hopping, Erber et al. 2010). In this study, the highest category of vegetable fiber intake was associated with a 22% lower risk of type 2 diabetes among men but not women (Hopping, Erber et al. 2010). These opposing and additive associations were replicated in a meta-regression analysis of 15 cross-sectional studies on several biomarkers including fasting glucose, HbA1c, and fructosamine (Livesey, Taylor et al. 2008).

Among short-term trials, high-fiber diets or fiber supplements generally improve glycemic control, insulin demand, and insulin sensitivity versus diets low in fiber (Weickert, Mohlig et al. 2006; Slavin 2008; Anderson, Baird et al. 2009). However, these benefits appear to be much stronger among individuals who are overweight or already have insulin resistance (Weickert, Mohlig et al. 2006; Slavin 2008; Anderson, Baird et al. 2009). In a meta-analysis of 6–12 trials comparing high-carbohydrate high-fiber diets to moderate-carbohydrate low-fiber diets (follow-up = 7–90 days) in participants with type 2 diabetes, the weighted mean fasting plasma glucose decreased by 14.3% (12 studies), whereas HbA1c decreased by 6% (6 studies) (Anderson, Randles et al. 2004). In a systematic review of three randomized trials among type 2 diabetics, 10.2 g of psyllium, a source of soluble fiber, significantly lowered fasting plasma glucose and HbA1c when given before meals (Bajorek and Morello 2011). Other studies utilizing euglycemic–hyperinsulinemic clamps have noted improvements in insulin sensitivity (Weickert and Pfeiffer 2008). Finally, in an observational study nested within a randomized trial from the Finnish Diabetes Prevention Study (intensive lifestyle counseling versus standard care), participants in the highest quartile of total fiber intake had a 62%

lower risk of type 2 diabetes over 4.1 years of follow up compared to those in the lowest quartile (Lindstrom, Peltonen et al. 2006).

Clearly, the most important mechanisms by which fiber can reduce the risk of type 2 diabetes is by trapping glucose and slowing its absorption in the gut, which lowers the glycemic index of the carbohydrate being digested (Livesey and Tagami 2009). However, another important mechanism is the increased production of short-chain fatty acids (acetate, propionate, and butyrate) by bacterial fermentation of soluble fiber and perhaps cereal fiber and resistant starches, which is thought to reduce hepatic glucose and lipid production (Weickert and Pfeiffer 2008). Cereal fiber may also enhance the secretion of glucagon-like peptide 1 that may reduce the amount of insulin required by individuals with impaired glucose metabolism (Slavin 2008). In addition, high intakes of cereal fiber have been positively associated with plasma adiponectin, which may improve insulin sensitivity by reducing triglyceride deposits in liver and skeletal muscle (Qi, Rimm et al. 2005). Similar to glycemic index, fiber intake has also been associated with lower levels of several soluble inflammatory markers. In a systematic review of seven cross-sectional studies, including the US National Health and Nutrition Examination Survey (Ajani, Ford et al. 2004), higher fiber intake was associated with lower levels of CRP (Butcher and Beckstrand 2010). Other studies have found inverse associations between fiber intake, IL-6, and TNF receptors (Ma, Hebert et al. 2008; Wannamethee, Whincup et al. 2009). And in a cross-sectional study of 902 women with type 2 diabetes from the Nurses' Health Study, cereal fiber intake was inversely associated with CRP and TNF-r2 (Qi, van Dam et al. 2006).

However, trials have not yet substantiated these findings. In a randomized trial of 158 overweight and obese participants, 7 or 14 g of psyllium was not successful in lowering CRP or IL-6 levels over 3 months (King, Mainous et al. 2008). Neither was a cereal fiber intervention using wheat bran successful in lowering CRP levels among 23 subjects with type 2 diabetes in a 3-month randomized crossover study (Jenkins, Kendall et al. 2002). These findings hint at confounding in the cross-sectional studies, perhaps by other dietary factors correlated with dietary fiber. Another explanation is simply that longer follow-up times and different types of fiber are required to observe an effect. A final potential mechanism is through changes in gut microflora, which promote the growth of organisms that modulate hepatic lipid and glucose synthesis. In a study of obese mice, the wheat fiber arabinoxylan restored populations of bifidobacteria, *Roseburia*, and *Bacteroides-Prevotella* species that were reduced following a high-fat diet (Neyrinck, Possemiers et al. 2011). These changes were also accompanied by weight loss and improvements in blood lipids.

Whole grains

Prior to the industrial revolution, all cereals were stone-milled and retained all the components of the grain (Cordain, Eaton et al. 2005). With the advent of steel roller milling and automated sifting in the late 19th century, large-scale refining of grains began—which significantly reduced the nutritional quality of grains (Cordain, Eaton et al. 2005). In the 1970s, Burkitt and Trowell were the first to note that African natives who consumed large quantities of unrefined whole plant foods had a very low prevalence of CHD, type 2 diabetes, and cancer (Burkitt and Trowell 1975). Since then, a number of epidemiological studies have added support to this hypothesis.

A whole grain kernel contains endosperm, germ, and bran, of which the proportions are unchanged by the processes of cracking, crushing, and flaking (Paul, Rokusek et al. 1996) [Figure 2.1]. However, the milling process removes germ and bran resulting in the loss of fiber, vitamins, minerals, lignans, resistant starch, phenolic compounds, and phytochemicals (Slavin, Martini et al. 1999). It is thought that these unique compounds confer health benefits.

Whole grains may be cooked and consumed either intact and unmodified (e.g., wheat berries, barley, and brown rice), or in foods made from milled whole grain flour (e.g., whole wheat pasta and whole wheat bread). Generally, intact grains have the lowest GI values among all forms of grains, followed by whole grain foods and refined grains. In 1999, the Food and Drug Association (FDA) established that for a health claim to be made about a product containing whole grains, 51% or more of the product by weight must be a whole grain ingredient (Ball, Greenhaff et al. 1996). However, not all whole grains provide the same health benefit, which makes it difficult to implement blanket public health recommendations about all whole grains. The lack of a universal definition and also reference methods for measuring whole grains content in foods also complicates matters.

Overweight and obesity

In epidemiologic studies, diets high in whole grains are associated with lower BMI and also abdominal obesity. In a systematic review published in 2008, whole grain intake or dietary patterns high in whole grains were associated with lower BMI and waist circumference among cross-sectional studies, prospective cohort studies, and randomized controlled trials—however, the majority of the evidence reviewed concerned observational studies (Williams, Grafenauer et al. 2008). In a separate meta-analysis of 15 cross-sectional studies, a comparison of the top versus the bottom category of whole grain intake was significantly associated with on average 0.63 kg/m² lower BMI, 2.7 cm lower waist circumference, and 0.023 units lower waist to hip ratio (Harland and Garton 2008). Importantly, a recent pooled analysis of 120,877 participants followed for over 20 years in the Nurses' Health Study, 12 years in the Nurses' Health Study II, and 20 in the Health Professionals Follow-up Study, strongly suggests that whole grains are important in preventing weight gain (Mozaffarian, Hao et al. 2011). In this study, participants gained on average 1.6 kg every 4 years, but for a 1 serving per day increase in whole grains participants gained 0.17 kg less (95% CI: −0.22 to −0.11, p < 0.0001) (Mozaffarian, Hao et al. 2011). In contrast, for a 1 serving per day increase in refined grains participants gained 0.18 kg (95% CI: 0.10–0.26) more (Mozaffarian, Hao et al. 2011). These changes were independent of other food intakes and confounders. And while these differences are clearly modest, it is important to note that whole grains are but one part of a healthy diet. When combined with other foods such as yogurt (−0.37 kg) and fruits (−0.22 kg), the cumulative impact is likely to be much larger (Mozaffarian, Hao et al. 2011). In contrast, with at least one exception (Pereira, Jacobs et al. 2002), trials comparing diets high in whole grains to refined grains have generally not found any significant difference in their effect on body weight (Melanson, Angelopoulos et al. 2006; Katcher, Legro et al. 2008; Williams, Grafenauer et al. 2008; Brownlee, Moore et al. 2010; Harris and Kris-Etherton 2010). However, several trials have found that whole grain intake tends to reduce abdominal adiposity and visceral fat (Katcher, Legro et al. 2008; Williams, Grafenauer et al. 2008; Brownlee, Moore et al. 2010; Harris and Kris-Etherton 2010; Kim, Kim et al. 2011). However, few trials have been performed and it is very difficult to draw conclusions from these data. Possible reasons for the discrepant results between observational studies and trials include (1) insufficient follow-up, (2) reduced compliance to the dietary intervention, (3) different sources and amounts of whole grains, (4) or confounding by other dietary or lifestyle factors in the observational studies.

The beneficial effects of whole grains on body weight are most likely mediated by fiber, which is contained in the bran. The high fiber and water content of whole grain foods makes them bulkier and less energy dense than their refined grain counterparts, which may help to promote satiety and reduce energy intake (Hu 2008). In addition, 20% to 50% of fiber in whole grain foods is viscous or soluble—which delays gastric emptying and intestinal absorption of nutrients, resulting in smaller peaks in plasma glucose and insulin (Koh-Banerjee and Rimm 2003). This should help to reduce hunger and satiety. The mechanism by which whole grains may reduce visceral and abdominal fat is unknown, but may be due to increased adipose tissue insulin sensitivity which decreases in lipoprotein lipase activity, fatty acid uptake and storage in visceral adipocytes (Harris and Kris-Etherton 2010).

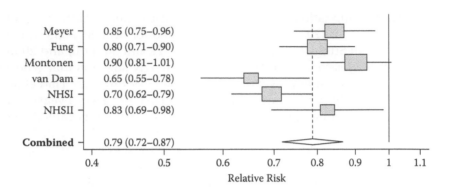

Figure 2.6 Meta-analysis of the relationship between a 2 serving/day increase in whole grain consumption and T2D among prospective cohort studies. (From de Munter, Hu et al. 2007. *PLoS Med* 4(8): e261.)

Type 2 diabetes

Among 5 prospective cohort studies included in a 2009 Cochrane review [Figure 2.6], whole-grain intake in the top versus the bottom category was associated with a pooled risk reduction for type 2 diabetes of 33% (RR = 0.67, 95% CO: 0.32–1.38) (Priebe, van Binsbergen et al. 2008). However, 36% of these studies did not adjust for other dietary and lifestyle factors, and only 3 studies adjusted for family history of diabetes and physical activity (Priebe, van Binsbergen et al. 2008). In a 2007 pooled analysis of 6 prospective cohort studies (combined n = 286,125, cases = 10,944, follow-up = 6–18 years), a two-serving per day increase in whole-grain intake was associated with a 21% (95% CI: 13%–28%) decreased risk of type 2 diabetes after adjusting for confounders and BMI (de Munter, Hu et al. 2007). In support of these findings, whole grain intake is inversely associated with blood glucose, insulin, and markers of glycemic control including C-peptide among several cross-sectional studies (Jensen, Koh-Banerjee et al. 2006; Harris and Kris-Etherton 2010). Also in a 2010 study that pooled results from the Nurses' Health Study, the Nurses Health Study II, and the Health Professionals Follow-up Study (combined n = 197,228, cases = 10,507, follow-up = 14–22 years), a comparison of the top versus the bottom quintile of whole grain intake was associated with a 27% lower risk of type 2 diabetes (RR = 0.73, 95% CI: 0.68–0.78) (Sun, Spiegelman et al. 2010). Studies examining the intake of specific whole grain foods report similar findings. In a prospective cohort study in 21,152 men with 19 years of follow-up, participants consuming at least 7 servings per week of whole grain breakfast cereals had 37% lower risk of type 2 diabetes (RR = 0.67, 95% CI: 0.55–0.72, p for trend <0.0001) versus those who did not consume breakfast cereal (Kochar, Djousse et al. 2007). This study adjusted for several possible confounders but did not adjust for total energy intake or other nutrients such as fiber or magnesium. Additional adjustment for BMI attenuated these results only slightly (RR = 0.69, 95% CI: 0.60–0.79) (Kochar, Djousse et al. 2007). In a pooled analysis of the Nurses' Health Study, Nurses Health Study II, and the Health Professionals Follow-up Study (combined n = 197,228, cases = 8148, mean follow-up = 14–22 years), a replacement of 50 g/per day (one-third of a serving) of white rice with brown rice was associated with a 16% risk reduction (RR = 0.84, 95% CI: 0.79–0.91), whereas replacement of white rice with an equivalent serving of whole grains was associated with a 36% risk reduction (RR = 0.64, 95% CI: 0.58–0.07) (Sun, Spiegelman et al. 2010). This study also found that bran but not germ intake was inversely associated with type 2 diabetes risk, which again supports a role for cereal fiber. This was also observed in an earlier study of the Nurses Health Study and Health Professionals' Follow-up Study (de Munter, Hu et al. 2007). Interestingly, markers of glycemic control were not appreciably different for equivalent intakes of bran and germ in a small cross-sectional sample of 938 participants from the Nurses Health Study II and the Health Professionals Follow-up Study (Jensen, Koh-Banerjee et al. 2006).

There have been no randomized trials of whole grain interventions on incident type 2 diabetes. However, many short-term trials of whole grain intake have been conducted with glucose, insulin, and markers of glycemic control as the outcomes. Pereira et al. conducted a 6-week cross-over trial in 11 hyperinsulinemic adults using either a whole or refined grain diet (twelve 30 g servings per day) and found a significant improvement in insulin sensitivity after the whole grain diet (Pereira, Jacobs et al. 2002). However, in a randomized trial of 266 overweight participants who routinely consume few whole grain products, no significant differences in fasting glucose and insulin were observed for diets containing 60 g of whole grains per day for 8 weeks, the same dietary treatment followed by 120 g of whole grains per day for 8 more weeks, and a control diet for 16 weeks (Brownlee, Moore et al. 2010). Another recent randomized trial also failed to find an effect of daily consumption of 3 portions of whole grain foods for 12 weeks on insulin sensitivity (Tighe, Duthie et al. 2010). In a randomized trial of a 210 individuals with type 2 diabetes, a diet high in whole grains and cereal fiber had a much smaller effect in lowering fasting glucose and HbA1c than did a low GL diet (Jenkins, Kendall et al. 2008).

The potential beneficial effects of whole grains on diabetes risk may be at least partly attributed to the fibrous bran. Bran contains many unique compounds that may favorably affect insulin sensitivity. For example, wheat bran contains antioxidant polyphenols and phytoestrogens, which may help to reduce inflammation, improve glycemia, and lower the risk of type 2 diabetes (Fardet 2010). In a 12-week randomized trial among 175 overweight individuals with impaired fasting glucose, a diet high in whole grains reduced CRP levels (–27%, p < 0.01) more than a complex healthy diet containing whole grains, bilberries, and fatty fish (–17%, p < 0.05) (de Mello, Schwab et al. 2011). In this study, whole grain bread intake had the strongest inverse association with CRP level among either diet (de Mello, Schwab et al. 2011). While other studies have observed inverse associations with CRP and TNF-R2 in some studies (Qi, van Dam et al. 2006), some—which include randomized trials—have not (Jensen, Koh-Banerjee et al. 2006; Brownlee, Moore et al. 2010; Tighe, Duthie et al. 2010). Thus, the impact of whole grains on inflammation is not entirely clear. Bran also contains magnesium, which improves insulin sensitivity by increasing tyrosine kinase activity at the level of the insulin receptor (Paolisso and Barbagallo 1997). Three meta-analyses of prospective studies indicate that increased magnesium intake is associated with a lower risk of type 2 diabetes (Larsson and Wolk 2007; Schulze, Schulz et al. 2007; Dong, Xun et al. 2011). These findings are partially supported by a meta-analysis of 9 short-term randomized trials (combined n = 370, follow-up = 4–16 weeks) of magnesium supplements among participants with type 2 diabetes, where an average dose of 360 mg/day produced significant albeit modest reductions in fasting glucose (–0.56 mmol/L, 95% CI: –1.01 to –0.01) but not HbA1c (Song, He et al. 2006). However, there was significant heterogeneity among these results, and the long-term effect of magnesium on glycemia are still unknown. Another component of bran that may help to reduce the development of type 2 diabetes are lignans, which have antioxidant and antiestrogenic effects (Bhathena and Velasquez 2002). Finally, whole grain intake is thought to alter the makeup of colonic bacteria—the significance of which is unclear. In a 3-week crossover study, daily intake of 48 g of whole grain breakfast cereal significantly increased fecal bifidobacteria and lactobacilli compared to wheat bran (Costabile, Klinder et al. 2008). This suggests that components in wheat germ may play a role in altering gut microflora.

Sugar-sweetened beverages

Dietary sugars may be either naturally occurring, or added to foods. Naturally occurring sugars such as fructose, sucrose, and lactose are those that are found in fruit, vegetables, dairy, and many grains. Added sugars are those that supplement foods during processing, preparation, and consumption. Food disappearance data indicates that over the past 40 years, added sugar—especially from high fructose corn syrup (HFCS)—has risen along with the prevalence of overweight and obesity in the United States (Gross, Li et al. 2004). Largely driving this trend is the dramatic increase in the consumption of sugar-sweetened beverages (SSB), which have become the largest source of added sugar in the US diet (Johnson, Appel et al. 2009). SSBs include carbonated soda, fruit drinks, sweetened tea, energy drinks, and other drinks that contain sweeteners such as sucrose, HFCS, or even fruit juice concentrates. In recent years, large epidemiological studies demonstrated relatively consistent relationships between intake of SSBs, long-term weight gain, and type 2 diabetes.

Overweight and obesity

Several systematic reviews indicate that intake of SSBs is associated with long-term weight gain and risk of overweight and obesity in both children and adults (Malik, Schulze et al. 2006; Vartanian, Schwartz et al. 2007; Malik, Willett et al. 2009; Hu and Malik 2010; Malik, Popkin et al. 2010). Associations are most consistent in large prospective cohort studies with long durations of follow-up that do not adjust for the potential mediating effect of total energy intake (Malik, Willett et al. 2009; Malik, Popkin et al. 2010). Total energy intake may be on the causal pathway between SSBs and weight gain, and so adjusting for total energy may remove any effect of SSB on body weight. This could explain some of the discrepancy between studies. Among the five largest prospective cohort studies in adults to date, daily SSB consumption was associated with weight gain. In a pooled analysis of the Nurses' Health Study (20 years of follow-up), the Nurses' Health Study II (12 years of follow-up), and the Health Professionals Follow-up Study (20 years of follow-up), 120,877 participants gained on average 1.6 kg every 4 years, but for a 1 serving per day increase in SSBs, they gained 0.45 kg more (95% CI: 0.38 to 0.53, p < 0.0001) (Mozaffarian, Hao et al. 2011). In contrast, for a 1 serving per day increase in diet soda, which does not contain energy, participants gained 0.05 kg less (95% CI: −0.10 to −0.01) (Mozaffarian, Hao et al. 2011). This was true after adjusting for other dietary and lifestyle factors, which reduces the possibility of confounding. Similar trends were observed in the Black Women's Health Study (*n* = 43,960, cases = 2713, follow-up = 6 years), where women who increased their intake from 1 or more servings per week to 1 or more servings per day gained the most weight, while those that decreased their intake gained the least weight (6.8 kg versus. 4.1 kg) (Palmer, Boggs et al. 2008). In the Singapore Chinese Health Study (*n* = 43,580, events = 2273, mean follow-up = 5.7 years), participants on average gained 0.10 kg, and participants in the highest category of SSB intake gained significantly more weight (0.53 kg) compared to those in the lowest category (p < 0.001) (Odegaard, Koh et al. 2010). Some smaller prospective studies have also been in agreement with these results, either in overall sample or among subgroup analyses (Malik, Schulze et al. 2006; Malik, Popkin et al. 2010).

In short-term trials which contrast SSBs to artificially sweetened beverages, SSB intake invariably leads to weight gain (Tordoff and Alleva 1990; Raben, Vasilaras et al. 2002). This is not surprising given that SSBs contain on average 150 calories and 36 g of sugar per 12 oz serving. If this extra energy intake is not balanced by a decreased energy intake at subsequent meals, weight gain will result (Malik, Popkin et al. 2010). Energy intake following consumption of liquid foods has been suggested to be higher than energy intake following consumption of isocaloric portions of solid food (DiMeglio and Mattes 2000). SSBs may therefore contribute to weight gain by interfering with the normal compensatory mechanism that leads to decreased intake of solid food (Malik, Popkin et al. 2010). While the exact mechanism behind this is unknown, several studies indicate that fructose intake is associated with lower levels of the satiating hormone leptin (Bray, Nielsen et al. 2004; Teff, Elliott et al. 2004; Teff, Grudziak et al. 2009). Fructose, which is a component of HFCS, also activates pathways of de novo lipogenesis, which could lead to increased numbers of adipocytes—especially visceral adipocytes—and a larger overall fat mass (Stanhope and Havel 2009; Stanhope, Schwarz et al. 2009; Malik, Popkin et al. 2010). It appears that well-designed, larger, and longer randomized trials will be needed to further our understanding on the possible extent to which SSB may impact weight gain, and whether SSB truly are unique in this regard compared to other beverages and to solid food.

Type 2 diabetes

In a recent meta-analysis of eight prospective cohort studies evaluating SSB intake and risk of type 2 diabetes (combined n = 310,819, cases = 15,043), individuals consuming 1–2 servings of SSBs per day had a 26% (RR = 1.26, 95% CI: 1.12–1.41) higher risk compared to those consuming none or <1 per month (Malik, Popkin et al. 2010) [Figure 2.7]. In this study, a 1 serving per day increase in SSB intake was associated with a 15% increase in risk (RR = 1.15, 95% CI: 1.11–1.20) (Malik, Popkin et al. 2010). Similar to studies of weight gain, these results were the most consistent among

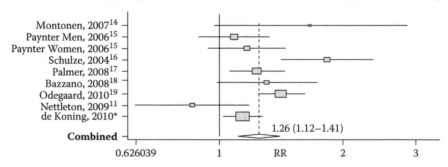

Figure 2.7 Meta-analysis of the relationship between sugar-sweetened beverage intake (comparison of extreme quantiles) and T2D among prospective cohort studies. (From Malik, Popkin et al. 2010.)

large studies with long follow-up that did not adjust for mediators such as total energy intake and BMI (Malik, Popkin et al. 2010). In analyses of the Nurses Health Study II (n = 92,749, cases = 741, mean follow-up = 8 years), those consuming one or more servings of SSBs per day had an 83% increased risk of developing type 2 diabetes compared to those consuming <1 per month (p trend < 0.001) (Schulze, Manson et al. 2004). These analyses were conducted after adjusting for other dietary factors, which could confound this relationship. Interestingly, adjusting for BMI attenuated the association by 50%, which suggests that much of this association is driven through changes in adiposity (Schulze, Manson et al. 2004). Interestingly, in the Health Professionals Follow-up Study, BMI adjustment had little impact on the overall association—however, adjusting for energy intake attenuated the association by half (de Koning, Malik et al. 2011). These findings suggest that body weight regulation may not be the most important mediator explaining the effect of SSB on type 2 diabetes risk. Direct physiological effects of SSB on glycemia, insulinemia, and other metabolic pathways need to be given careful attention in future studies.

Short-term trials have provided valuable insight into potential mechanisms by which SSBs can elevate the risk of type 2 diabetes independent of BMI. This may be related to large quantities of rapidly absorbable carbohydrates present in SSBs, such as HFCS (Schulze, Manson et al. 2004). Rapid and dramatic spikes in blood glucose and insulin accompany SSB intake, and combined with the high prevalence of their consumption, contribute to a very high dietary GL (Janssens, Shapira et al. 1999). As mentioned earlier, high GI/GL diets are thought to stimulate appetite and weight gain through rapid and transient insulinemia (Ludwig 2002). They also may lead to glucose intolerance and insulin resistance and type 2 diabetes, particularly among those who are already overweight (Ludwig 2002).

Other unique pro-diabetic mechanisms may be associated with SSB intake. First, the increased GI/GL associated with SSBs likely leads to increased levels of soluble inflammatory factors such as CRP. This has been seen in several observational studies (Qi, van Dam et al. 2006) and trials (Wolever, Gibbs et al. 2008). However, up until recently, there have been no trials that have specifically tested the health effects of SSBs. In a 3-week crossover trial of 29 participants randomized to one of 5 SSB interventions (600 mL per day of moderate [40 g] fructose, high [80 g] fructose, moderate [40 g] glucose, high [80 g] glucose, high [80 g] sucrose) or dietary advice to reduce fructose, CRP levels rose significantly in all beverage interventions but the greatest increase was among those receiving the high fructose treatment (Aeberli, Gerber et al. 2011). In a separate 10-week intervention study comparing the effects of sucrose and artificially sweeteners on markers of inflammation, serum levels of haptoglobin, transferring, and CRP were significantly elevated in the sucrose group compared to the artificial sweetener group (Sorensen, Raben et al. 2005). Among observational studies, in a nested case control study of type 2 diabetes in the Nurses Health Study, a dietary pattern high in SSBs was associated with higher levels of several inflammatory factors including TNF-r2, IL-6, and CRP which explained the greatest proportion type 2 diabetes risk (Schulze, Hoffmann et al. 2005). Second, advanced glycation end products found in the caramel coloring of cola beverages may contribute to increased diabetes risk, as they are associated with insulin resistance in animal models (Vlassara, Cai et al. 2002). Third, fructose that is present in large quantities in HFCS may exert additional adverse metabolic effects. Fructose stimulates hepatic de novo lipogenesis, which leads to high triglycerides, low HDL cholesterol, small dense LDL, insulin resistance (Bray 2007). SSBs may also lead to an increase in highly insulin resistant visceral fat, and while this hypothesis has recently been supported by a cross-sectional observational study (Odegaard, Choh et al. 2012) and a small experimental study (Maersk, Belza et al. 2012), more research is certainly required.

Insulin index and load

While glycemic index (GI), glycemic load (GL), and the postprandial glycemia associated with them have been comprehensively studied for relations with overweight, obesity, and type 2 diabetes, dietary insulin response has not been explored. This is because, in general, postprandial elevations in insulin closely follow glucose. However, there are some exceptions. Blood insulin levels increase when protein or fat is added to a carbohydrate-rich meal, whereas glucose levels do not change or may even decrease (Collier, McLean et al. 1984; Nuttall, Mooradian et al. 1984). This effect is potentiated by insulinotropic factors including fructose, certain amino acids, fatty acids, gastric inhibitory protein (GIP), and glucagon-like protein 1 (Holt, Miller et al. 1997; Frid, Nilsson et al. 2005). Increased insulin demand by the consumption of highly insulinemic foods may accelerate beta cell failure, leading to type 2 diabetes (Grill and Bjorklund 2009). Insulin response appears to be an extremely important area of study in diabetes epidemiology, given that genome-wide scans of type 2 diabetes related-loci identified far more SNPs in genes related to insulin secretion than insulin resistance (Billings and Florez 2010).

In 1997, Holt and colleagues developed the food insulin index (II) using methods similar to those used by Jenkins et al. to create the glycemic index (Holt, Miller et al. 1997). The II is derived by expressing postprandial blood insulin response to a given food as a percentage of response to white bread (Holt, Miller et al. 1997). Unlike the GI, however, which is determined among foods with identical carbohydrate content, the II is determined among isoenergetic (1000 kcal) portions of food. This is because insulinemia is affected not only by carbohydrate, but protein and fat as well. In particular, high protein foods such as beef have the highest II relative to glucose response (Jenkins, Wolever et al. 1981; Bao, de Jong et al. 2009). Insulin load (IL) is calculated as the product of II and energy content and, like GL, takes into account both carbohydrate quality and quantity (Bao, de Jong et al. 2009).

Similar to GI and GL, II and IL can be used to predict insulin response to complex meals. For II, this is calculated as the energy-weighted average of all II values in a meal. For IL, it is simply the sum of all food ILs (II * calories). Meal IL shows great promise in accurately predicting postprandial insulin response. In a recent study where 13 different isoenergetic meals were administered to 21 men and women, IL had the strongest correlation ($r = 0.8$, $p < 0.01$) with postprandial insulin AUC compared to GL ($r = 0.7$, $p = 0.01$), total fat intake ($r = -0.6$, $p = 0.03$), protein ($r \sim -0.1$, $p = 0.88$), and carbohydrate ($r = 0.5$, $p = 0.06$) (Bao, de Jong et al. 2009).

However, few studies have utilized II/IL, perhaps because of the scarcity of data on insulin response of foods and complex meals. To date, no studies have examined associations with overweight, obesity, or type 2 diabetes. However, in a cross-sectional study of 4002 participants from the Nurses' Health Study and the Health Professionals Follow-up Study, II and IL were tested for their associations with fasting concentrations of plasma C-peptide, HbA1c, HDL cholesterol, LDL cholesterol, triglycerides, C-reactive protein (CRP), and interleukin-6 (IL-6). Participants in the top quintile of II/IL had approximately 26% higher triglyceride concentrations than participants in the lowest quintile (P for trend < 0.0001). This association was significantly stronger among obese participants (72%; p for trend = 0.01). Dietary II/IL was also inversely associated with HDL cholesterol in obese participants (–18%; P for trend = 0.03). Two pooled analyses of the Nurses Health Study and the Health Professionals Follow-up Study found no significant overall associations between II and pancreatic cancer (Bao, Nimptsch et al. 2011), prostate cancer (Nimptsch, Kenfield et al. 2011), and colorectal cancer (Bao, Nimptsch et al. 2011) incidence—all of which are common cancers believed to be stimulated by high insulin levels. However, the authors did find a significant association between II/IL and pancreatic cancer (Bao, Nimptsch et al. 2011) incidence among individuals who were overweight or obese (Bao, Nimptsch et al. 2011). Further studies are necessary to determine whether the II and IL provide additional predictive power on type 2 diabetes over GI and GL.

Summary and public health implications

Carbohydrate intake has risen dramatically in the United States over the past 50 years, and is mostly due to higher intake of highly processed, low-quality carbohydrates. These trends may have been fueled by public health messages based on the misguided belief that carbohydrates are homogenous and either uniformly beneficial or innocuous, and therefore should be consumed in place of "dangerous" dietary fat. Combined with the rise of food processing and carbohydrate refinement on a massive scale, these trends in consumption patterns may have had negative consequences for the prevalence of overweight, obesity, and type 2 diabetes in industrialized countries.

Carbohydrates are not homogenous entities, nor are they innocuous. The simple versus complex labeling system of carbohydrate should be abandoned because it does not address health concerns, which are the most important considerations. Total carbohydrate intake, as measured by the proportion of energy provided by total carbohydrate, is a relatively insensitive metric that is not associated with overweight, obesity, or type 2 diabetes because, across individual in the population, it is a blend of healthy and unhealthy carbohydrates—and its association with health outcomes is likely obscured by the reciprocal contributions of dietary fats and proteins. Glycemic index, glycemic load, insulin index, and insulin load are experimentally derived, highly specific carbohydrate classification systems that were designed to identify carbohydrates by their immediate impact on glycemia and insulinemia. However, food databases for GI/GL or II/IL are not comprehensive, food values vary enormously, and using them to plan meals can be cumbersome. In contrast, fiber content is a simple metric that is highly predictive of health outcomes and is also correlated with GI/GL. Similarly, whole and intact grains are correlated with both fiber and GI/GL, and contain important health promoting compounds that isolated fiber does not. Sugar-sweetened beverages are important because of their extremely high intake in Western countries, their strong acute effect on glycemia and insulinemia, and their relatively consistent positive association with risk of type 2 diabetes.

The bottom line is that carbohydrate usually provides the majority of food energy in the human diet, and therefore an improvement in the quality of dietary carbohydrate should have significant health benefits. Public health messages for population-wide reductions in total carbohydrate intake can be achieved by recommending the replacement of some dietary carbohydrate with healthy vegetable sources of protein and fats (e.g., legumes and nuts). This approach will help to lower dietary GI/GL. However, to make the largest impact on GI/GL as well to increase the intakes of insoluble fiber, soluble fiber and resistant starch, foods high in refined grains (e.g., white bread) and easily digestible starches (e.g., tubers), should be replaced with whole grains (e.g., whole wheat breads, whole breakfast cereals), legumes, vegetables, and fruits. A further recommendation must center on the replacement of sugar-sweetened beverages with healthier alternatives such as milk, water, coffee, or tea. Artificially sweetened beverages may be useful alternatives to SSBs;

however, controversy still surrounds their use, as they are occasionally associated with adverse health outcomes. These matters are discussed in more detail in Chapter 7.

References

Abete, I., A. Astrup et al. (2010). "Obesity and the metabolic syndrome: Role of different dietary macronutrient distribution patterns and specific nutritional components on weight loss and maintenance." *Nutr Rev* **68**(4): 214–231.

Aeberli, I., P. A. Gerber et al. (2011). "Low to moderate sugar-sweetened beverage consumption impairs glucose and lipid metabolism and promotes inflammation in healthy young men: A randomized controlled trial." *Am J Clin Nutr* **94**(2): 479–485.

Ajani, U. A., E. S. Ford et al. (2004). "Dietary fiber and C-reactive protein: Findings from national health and nutrition examination survey data." *J Nutr* **134**(5): 1181–1185.

Anderson, J. W., P. Baird et al. (2009). "Health benefits of dietary fiber." *Nutr Rev* **67**(4): 188–205.

Anderson, J. W., K. M. Randles et al. (2004). "Carbohydrate and fiber recommendations for individuals with diabetes: A quantitative assessment and meta-analysis of the evidence." *J Am Coll Nutr* **23**(1): 5–17.

Atkins, R. C. (2002). *Dr Atkins' New Diet Revolution, Revised Edition*. Plymouth, Rowman and Littlefield.

Atkinson, F. S., K. Foster-Powell et al. (2008). "International tables of glycemic index and glycemic load values: 2008." *Diabetes Care* **31**(12): 2281–2283.

Bajorek, S. A. and C. M. Morello (2011). "Effects of dietary fiber and low glycemic index diet on glucose control in subjects with type 2 diabetes mellitus." *Ann Pharmacother* **44**(11): 1786–1792.

Ball, D., P. L. Greenhaff et al. (1996). "The acute reversal of a diet-induced metabolic acidosis does not restore endurance capacity during high-intensity exercise in man." *Eur J Appl Physiol Occup Physiol* **73**(1–2): 105–112.

Bantle, J. P., J. E. Swanson et al. (1993). "Metabolic effects of dietary sucrose in type II diabetic subjects." *Diabetes Care* **16**(9): 1301–1305.

Bao, J., V. de Jong et al. (2009). "Food insulin index: Physiologic basis for predicting insulin demand evoked by composite meals." *Am J Clin Nutr* **90**(4): 986–992.

Bao, Y., K. Nimptsch et al. (2011a). "Dietary insulin load, dietary insulin index, and colorectal cancer." *Cancer Epidemiol Biomarkers Prev* **19**(12): 3020–3026.

Bao, Y., K. Nimptsch et al. (2011b). "Dietary insulin load, dietary insulin index, and risk of pancreatic cancer." *Am J Clin Nutr* **94**(3): 862–868.

Barclay, A. W., V. M. Flood et al. (2007). "Glycemic index, dietary fiber, and risk of type 2 diabetes in a cohort of older Australians." *Diabetes Care* **30**(11): 2811–2813.

Barclay, A. W., P. Petocz et al. (2008). "Glycemic index, glycemic load, and chronic disease risk—a meta-analysis of observational studies." *Am J Clin Nutr* **87**(3): 627–637.

Behall, K. M., D. J. Scholfield et al. (1988). "Effect of starch structure on glucose and insulin responses in adults." *Am J Clin Nutr* **47**(3): 428–432.

Bhathena, S. J. and M. T. Velasquez (2002). "Beneficial role of dietary phytoestrogens in obesity and diabetes." *Am J Clin Nutr* **76**(6): 1191–1201.

Billings, L. K. and J. C. Florez (2010). "The genetics of type 2 diabetes: What have we learned from GWAS?" *Ann N Y Acad Sci* **1212**: 59–77.

Bingham, S., R. Luben et al. (2007). "Epidemiologic assessment of sugars consumption using biomarkers: Comparisons of obese and nonobese individuals in the European prospective investigation of cancer Norfolk." *Cancer Epidemiol Biomarkers Prev* **16**(8): 1651–1654.

Bouche, C., S. W. Rizkalla et al. (2002). "Five-week, low-glycemic index diet decreases total fat mass and improves plasma lipid profile in moderately overweight nondiabetic men." *Diabetes Care* **25**(5): 822–828.

Boyle, J. P., T. J. Thompson et al. (2010). "Projection of the year 2050 burden of diabetes in the US adult population: Dynamic modeling of incidence, mortality, and prediabetes prevalence." *Popul Health Metr* **8**: 29.

Brand-Miller, J., S. Hayne et al. (2003). "Low-glycemic index diets in the management of diabetes: A meta-analysis of randomized controlled trials." *Diabetes Care* **26**(8): 2261–2267.

Bray, G. A. (2007). "How bad is fructose?" *Am J Clin Nutr* **86**(4): 895–896.

Bray, G. A., S. J. Nielsen et al. (2004). "Consumption of high-fructose corn syrup in beverages may play a role in the epidemic of obesity." *Am J Clin Nutr* **79**(4): 537–543.

Brehm, B. J., B. L. Lattin et al. (2009). "One-year comparison of a high-monounsaturated fat diet with a high-carbohydrate diet in type 2 diabetes." *Diabetes Care* **32**(2): 215–220.

Brenner, B. M., E. V. Lawler et al. (1996). "The hyperfiltration theory: A paradigm shift in nephrology." *Kidney Int* **49**(6): 1774–1777.

Brownlee, I. A., C. Moore et al. (2010). "Markers of cardiovascular risk are not changed by increased whole-grain intake: The WHOLEheart study, a randomised, controlled dietary intervention." *Br J Nutr* **104**(1): 125–134.

Brownlee, M. (2001). "Biochemistry and molecular cell biology of diabetic complications." *Nature* **414**(6865): 813–820.

Brunner, E., D. Stallone et al. (2001). "Dietary assessment in Whitehall II: Comparison of 7 d diet diary and food-frequency questionnaire and validity against biomarkers." *Br J Nutr* **86**(3): 405–414.

Brynes, A. E. and G. S. Frost (2007). "Increased sucrose intake is not associated with a change in glucose or insulin sensitivity in people with type 2 diabetes." *Int J Food Sci Nutr* **58**(8): 644–651.

Burkitt, D. and H. Trowell (1975). *Refined Carbohydrate Foods and Disease: Some Implications PF Dietary Fiber.* London, United Kingdom, Academic Press.

Butcher, J. L. and R. L. Beckstrand (2010). "Fiber's impact on high-sensitivity C-reactive protein levels in cardiovascular disease." *J Am Acad Nurse Pract* **22**(11): 566–572.

Collier, G., A. McLean et al. (1984). "Effect of co-ingestion of fat on the metabolic responses to slowly and rapidly absorbed carbohydrates." *Diabetologia* **26**(1): 50–54.

Cordain, L., S. B. Eaton et al. (2005). "Origins and evolution of the Western diet: Health implications for the 21st century." *Am J Clin Nutr* **81**(2): 341–354.

Costabile, A., A. Klinder et al. (2008). "Whole-grain wheat breakfast cereal has a prebiotic effect on the human gut microbiota: A double-blind, placebo-controlled, crossover study." *Br J Nutr* **99**(1): 110–120.

Curhan, G. C., W. C. Willett et al. (1993). "A prospective study of dietary calcium and other nutrients and the risk of symptomatic kidney stones." *N Engl J Med* **328**(12): 833–838.

Davis, N. J., N. Tomuta et al. (2009). "Comparative study of the effects of a 1-year dietary intervention of a low-carbohydrate diet versus a low-fat diet on weight and glycemic control in type 2 diabetes." *Diabetes Care* **32**(7): 1147–1152.

de Koning, L. (2011). Low-carbohydrate diets and risk of coronary heart disease in men.

de Koning, L., T. T. Fung et al. (2011). "Low-carbohydrate diet scores and risk of type 2 diabetes in men." *Am J Clin Nutr* **93**(4): 844–850.

de Koning, L., V. S. Malik et al. (2011). "Sugar-sweetened and artificially sweetened beverage consumption and risk of type 2 diabetes in men." *Am J Clin Nutr* **93**(6): 1321–1327.

de Mello, V. D., U. Schwab et al. (2011). "A diet high in fatty fish, bilberries and wholegrain products improves markers of endothelial function and inflammation in individuals with impaired glucose metabolism in a randomised controlled trial: The Sysdimet study." *Diabetologia* **54**(11): 2755–2767.

de Munter, J. S., F. B. Hu et al. (2007). "Whole grain, bran, and germ intake and risk of type 2 diabetes: A prospective cohort study and systematic review." *PLoS Med* **4**(8): e261.

De Natale, C., G. Annuzzi et al. (2009). "Effects of a plant-based high-carbohydrate/high-fiber diet versus high-monounsaturated fat/low-carbohydrate diet on postprandial lipids in type 2 diabetic patients." *Diabetes Care* **32**(12): 2168–2173.

DiMeglio, D. P. and R. D. Mattes (2000). "Liquid versus solid carbohydrate: Effects on food intake and body weight." *Int J Obes Relat Metab Disord* **24**(6): 794–800.

Doebley, J. (2004). "The genetics of maize evolution." *Annu Rev Genet* **38**: 37–59.

Dong, J. Y., P. Xun et al. (2011). "Magnesium intake and risk of type 2 diabetes: Meta-analysis of prospective cohort studies." *Diabetes Care* **34**(9): 2116–2122.

Du, H., A. D. van der et al. (2010). "Dietary fiber and subsequent changes in body weight and waist circumference in European men and women." *Am J Clin Nutr* **91**(2): 329–336.

Du, H., A. D. van der et al. (2009). "Dietary glycaemic index, glycaemic load and subsequent changes of weight and waist circumference in European men and women." *Int J Obes (Lond)* **33**(11): 1280–1288.

Du, S., B. Lu et al. (2002). "A new stage of the nutrition transition in China." *Public Health Nutr* **5**(1 A): 169–174.

Duffey, K. J. and B. M. Popkin (2008). "High-fructose corn syrup: Is this what's for dinner?" *Am J Clin Nutr* **88**(6): 1722S–1732S.

Eaton, S. B. (2006). "The ancestral human diet: What was it and should it be a paradigm for contemporary nutrition?" *Proc Nutr Soc* **65**(1): 1–6.

Eaton, S. B. and S. B. Eaton, (2000). "Paleolithic vs. modern diets—selected pathophysiological implications." *Eur J Nutr* **39**(2): 67–70.

Ebbeling, C. B., M. M. Leidig et al. (2007). "Effects of a low-glycemic load vs low-fat diet in obese young adults: A randomized trial." *Jama* **297**(19): 2092–2102.

Ebbeling, C. B., M. M. Leidig et al. (2003). "A reduced-glycemic load diet in the treatment of adolescent obesity." *Arch Pediatr Adolesc Med* **157**(8): 773–779.

Ebbeling, C. B., M. M. Leidig et al. (2005). "Effects of an ad libitum low-glycemic load diet on cardiovascular disease risk factors in obese young adults." *Am J Clin Nutr* **81**(5): 976–982.

Esfahani, A., J. M. Wong et al. (2009). "The glycemic index: Physiological significance." *J Am Coll Nutr* **28**(suppl.): 439S–445S.

Esposito, K., F. Nappo et al. (2002). "Inflammatory cytokine concentrations are
acutely increased by hyperglycemia in humans: Role of oxidative stress."
Circulation **106**(16): 2067–2072.

Fardet, A. (2010). "New hypotheses for the health-protective mechanisms of
whole-grain cereals: What is beyond fibre?" *Nutr Res Rev* **23**(1): 65–134.

Food and Agriculture Organization of the United Nations. (2009). "FAOSTAT:
World Production of barley, maize, millett, mixed grain, rice, roots and
tubers, rye and wheat," from http://faostat.fao.org.

Food and Nutrition Board (2002/2005). Dietary Reference Intakes for Energy, C.,
Fiber, Fat, Fatty Acids, Cholesterol, Protein, and Amino Acids. Washington,
D.C.: The National Academies Press, p. 769.

Frid, A. H., M. Nilsson et al. (2005). "Effect of whey on blood glucose and insulin
responses to composite breakfast and lunch meals in type 2 diabetic subjects." *Am J Clin Nutr* **82**(1): 69–75.

Gaesser, G. A. (2007). "Carbohydrate quantity and quality in relation to body mass
index." *J Am Diet Assoc* **107**(10): 1768–1780.

Grill, V. and A. Bjorklund (2009). "Impact of metabolic abnormalities for beta
cell function: Clinical significance and underlying mechanisms." *Mol Cell
Endocrinol* **297**(1–2): 86–92.

Gross, L. S., L. Li et al. (2004). "Increased consumption of refined carbohydrates
and the epidemic of type 2 diabetes in the United States: An ecologic assessment." *Am J Clin Nutr* **79**(5): 774–779.

Halton, T. L. and F. B. Hu (2004). "The effects of high protein diets on thermogenesis, satiety and weight loss: A critical review." *J Am Coll Nutr* **23**(5): 373–385.

Halton, T. L., S. Liu et al. (2008). "Low-carbohydrate-diet score and risk of type 2
diabetes in women." *Am J Clin Nutr* **87**(2): 339–346.

Halton, T. L., W. C. Willett et al. (2006). "Low-carbohydrate-diet score and the risk
of coronary heart disease in women." *N Engl J Med* **355**(19): 1991–2002.

Hare-Bruun, H., A. Flint et al. (2006). "Glycemic index and glycemic load in relation to changes in body weight, body fat distribution, and body composition
in adult Danes." *Am J Clin Nutr* **84**(4): 871–879; quiz 952–873.

Harland, J. I. and L. E. Garton (2008). "Whole-grain intake as a marker of healthy
body weight and adiposity." *Public Health Nutr* **11**(6): 554–563.

Harris, K. A. and P. M. Kris-Etherton (2010). "Effects of whole grains on coronary
heart disease risk." *Curr Atheroscler Rep* **12**(6): 368–376.

Hession, M., C. Rolland et al. (2009). "Systematic review of randomized controlled
trials of low-carbohydrate vs. low-fat/low-calorie diets in the management
of obesity and its comorbidities." *Obes Rev* **10**(1): 36–50.

Hiatt, R. A., B. Ettinger et al. (1996). "Randomized controlled trial of a low animal
protein, high fiber diet in the prevention of recurrent calcium oxalate kidney
stones." *Am J Epidemiol* **144**(1): 25–33.

Higgins, J. A., M. R. Jackman et al. (2010). "Resistant starch and exercise independently attenuate weight regain on a high fat diet in a rat model of obesity."
Nutr Metab (Lond) **8**: 49.

Hite, A. H., R. D. Feinman et al. (2010). "In the face of contradictory evidence: Report
of the Dietary Guidelines for Americans Committee." *Nutrition* **26**(10): 915–924.

Holt, S. H., J. C. Miller et al. (1997). "An insulin index of foods: The insulin demand generated by 1000-kJ portions of common foods." *Am J Clin Nutr* **66**(5): 1264–1276.

Hopping, B. N., E. Erber et al. (2010). "Dietary fiber, magnesium, and glycemic load alter risk of type 2 diabetes in a multiethnic cohort in Hawaii." *J Nutr* **140**(1): 68–74.

Hotamisligil, G. S. (2006). "Inflammation and metabolic disorders." *Nature* **444**(7121): 860–867.

Howarth, N. C., E. Saltzman et al. (2001). "Dietary fiber and weight regulation." *Nutr Rev* **59**(5): 129–139.

Hu, F. B. (2008). *Obesity Epidemiology*. New York, Oxford University Press.

Hu, F. B. (2010). "Are refined carbohydrates worse than saturated fat?" *Am J Clin Nutr* **91**(6): 1541–1542.

Hu, F. B. and V. S. Malik (2010). "Sugar-sweetened beverages and risk of obesity and type 2 diabetes: Epidemiologic evidence." *Physiol Behav* **100**(1): 47–54.

Janket, S. J., J. E. Manson et al. (2003). "A prospective study of sugar intake and risk of type 2 diabetes in women." *Diabetes Care* **26**(4): 1008–1015.

Janssens, J. P., N. Shapira et al. (1999). "Effects of soft drink and table beer consumption on insulin response in normal teenagers and carbohydrate drink in youngsters." *Eur J Cancer Prev* **8**(4): 289–295.

Jenkins, D. J., C. W. Kendall et al. (2002). "Effect of wheat bran on glycemic control and risk factors for cardiovascular disease in type 2 diabetes." *Diabetes Care* **25**(9): 1522–1528.

Jenkins, D. J., C. W. Kendall et al. (2008). "Effect of a low-glycemic index or a high

Jenkins, D. J., T. M. Wolever et al. (1981). "Glycemic index of foods: A physiological basis for carbohydrate exchange." *Am J Clin Nutr* **34**(3): 362–366.

Jenkins, D. J., J. M. Wong et al. (2009). "The effect of a plant-based low-carbohydrate ("Eco-Atkins") diet on body weight and blood lipid concentrations in hyperlipidemic subjects." *Arch Intern Med* **169**(11): 1046–1054.

Jensen, M. K., P. Koh-Banerjee et al. (2006). "Whole grains, bran, and germ in relation to homocysteine and markers of glycemic control, lipids, and inflammation 1." *Am J Clin Nutr* **83**(2): 275–283.

Johnson, R. K., L. J. Appel et al. (2009). "Dietary sugars intake and cardiovascular health: A scientific statement from the American Heart Association." *Circulation* **120**(11): 1011–1020.

Katcher, H. I., R. S. Legro et al. (2008). "The effects of a whole grain-enriched hypocaloric diet on cardiovascular disease risk factors in men and women with metabolic syndrome." *Am J Clin Nutr* **87**(1): 79–90.

Kelly, S., G. Frost et al. (2004). "Low glycaemic index diets for coronary heart disease." *Cochrane Database Syst Rev*(4): CD004467.

Kim, T. H., E. K. Kim et al. (2011). "Intake of brown rice lees reduces waist circumference and improves metabolic parameters in type 2 diabetes." *Nutr Res* **31**(2). 131–138.

King, D. E., A. G. Mainous et al. (2008). "Effect of psyllium fiber supplementation on C-reactive protein: The trial to reduce inflammatory markers (TRIM)." *Ann Fam Med* **6**(2): 100–106.

Kochar, J., L. Djousse et al. (2007). "Breakfast cereals and risk of type 2 diabetes in the Physicians' Health Study I." *Obesity (Silver Spring)* **15**(12): 3039–3044.

Koh-Banerjee, P., N. F. Chu et al. (2003). "Prospective study of the association of changes in dietary intake, physical activity, alcohol consumption, and smoking with 9-y gain in waist circumference among 16 587 US men." *Am J Clin Nutr* **78**(4): 719–727.

Koh-Banerjee, P., M. Franz et al. (2004). "Changes in whole-grain, bran, and cereal fiber consumption in relation to 8-y weight gain among men." *Am J Clin Nutr* **80**(5): 1237–1245.

Koh-Banerjee, P. and E. B. Rimm (2003). "Whole grain consumption and weight gain: A review of the epidemiological evidence, potential mechanisms and opportunities for future research." *Proc Nutr Soc* **62**(1): 25–29.

Konner, M. and S. B. Eaton (2011). "Paleolithic nutrition: Twenty-five years later." *Nutr Clin Pract* **25**(6): 594–602.

Krishnan, S., L. Rosenberg et al. (2007). "Glycemic index, glycemic load, and cereal fiber intake and risk of type 2 diabetes in US black women." *Arch Intern Med* **167**(21): 2304–2309.

Krog-Mikkelsen, I., B. Sloth et al. (2011). "A low glycemic index diet does not affect postprandial energy metabolism but decreases postprandial insulinemia and increases fullness ratings in healthy women." *J Nutr* **141**(9): 1679–1684.

Larsson, S. C. and A. Wolk (2007). "Magnesium intake and risk of type 2 diabetes: A meta-analysis." *J Intern Med* **262**(2): 208–214.

Lev-Yadun, S., A. Gopher et al. (2000). "Archaeology. The cradle of agriculture." *Science* **288**(5471): 1602–1603.

Levitan, E. B., N. R. Cook et al. (2008). "Dietary glycemic index, dietary glycemic load, blood lipids, and C-reactive protein." *Metabolism* **57**(3): 437–443.

Lindstrom, J., M. Peltonen et al. (2006). "High-fibre, low-fat diet predicts long-term weight loss and decreased type 2 diabetes risk: The Finnish Diabetes Prevention Study." *Diabetologia* **49**(5): 912–920.

Liu, S., J. E. Manson et al. (2002). "Relation between a diet with a high glycemic load and plasma concentrations of high-sensitivity C-reactive protein in middle-aged women." *Am J Clin Nutr* **75**(3): 492–498.

Liu, S., W. C. Willett et al. (2003). "Relation between changes in intakes of dietary fiber and grain products and changes in weight and development of obesity among middle-aged women." *Am J Clin Nutr* **78**(5): 920–927.

Livesey, G. and H. Tagami (2009). "Interventions to lower the glycemic response to carbohydrate foods with a low-viscosity fiber (resistant maltodextrin): Meta-analysis of randomized controlled trials." *Am J Clin Nutr* **89**(1): 114–125.

Livesey, G., R. Taylor et al. (2008). "Glycemic response and health—a systematic review and meta-analysis: Relations between dietary glycemic properties and health outcomes." *Am J Clin Nutr* **87**(1): 258S–268S.

Ludwig, D. S. (2000). "Dietary glycemic index and obesity." *J Nutr* **130**(2S Suppl): 280S–283S.

Ludwig, D. S. (2002). "The glycemic index: Physiological mechanisms relating to obesity, diabetes, and cardiovascular disease." *JAMA* **287**(18): 2414–2423.

Ludwig, D. S., M. A. Pereira et al. (1999). "Dietary fiber, weight gain, and cardiovascular disease risk factors in young adults." *Jama* **282**(16): 1539–1546.

Ma, Y., J. R. Hebert et al. (2008). "Association between dietary fiber and markers of systemic inflammation in the Women's Health Initiative Observational Study." *Nutrition* **24**(10): 941–949.

Ma, Y., B. Olendzki et al. (2005). "Association between dietary carbohydrates and body weight." *Am J Epidemiol* **161**(4): 359–367.

Maersk, M., A. Belza et al. (2012). "Sucrose-sweetened beverages increase fat storage in the liver, muscle, and visceral fat depot: A 6-mo randomized intervention study." *Am J Clin Nutr* **95**(2): 283–289.

Malik, V. S. and F. B. Hu (2007). "Popular weight-loss diets: From evidence to practice." *Nat Clin Pract Cardiovasc Med* **4**(1): 34–41.

Malik, V. S., B. M. Popkin et al. (2010a). "Sugar-sweetened beverages, obesity, type 2 diabetes mellitus, and cardiovascular disease risk." *Circulation* **121**(11): 1356–1364.

Malik, V. S., B. M. Popkin et al. (2010b). "Sugar-sweetened beverages and risk of metabolic syndrome and type 2 diabetes: A meta-analysis." *Diabetes Care* **33**(11): 2477–2483.

Malik, V. S., M. B. Schulze et al. (2006). "Intake of sugar-sweetened beverages and weight gain: A systematic review." *Am J Clin Nutr* **84**(2): 274–288.

Malik, V. S., W. C. Willett et al. (2009). "Sugar-sweetened beverages and BMI in children and adolescents: Reanalyses of a meta-analysis." *Am J Clin Nutr* **89**(1): 438–439; author reply 439–440.

McMillan-Price, J., P. Petocz et al. (2006). "Comparison of 4 diets of varying glycemic load on weight loss and cardiovascular risk reduction in overweight and obese young adults: A randomized controlled trial." *Arch Intern Med* **166**(14): 1466–1475.

Melanson, K. J., T. J. Angelopoulos et al. (2006). "Consumption of whole-grain cereals during weight loss: Effects on dietary quality, dietary fiber, magnesium, vitamin B-6, and obesity." *J Am Diet Assoc* **106**(9): 1380–1388; quiz 1389–1390.

Mensink, R. P., P. L. Zock et al. (2003). "Effects of dietary fatty acids and carbohydrates on the ratio of serum total to HDL cholesterol and on serum lipids and apolipoproteins: A meta-analysis of 60 controlled trials." *Am J Clin Nutr* **77**(5): 1146–1155.

Meyer, K. A., L. H. Kushi et al. (2000). "Carbohydrates, dietary fiber, and incident type 2 diabetes in older women." *Am J Clin Nutr* **71**(4): 921–930.

Miller, D. S. and P. A. Judd (1984). "The metabolisable energy value of foods." *J Sci Food Agric* **35**(1): 111–116.

Miller, J. C. (1994). "Importance of glycemic index in diabetes." *Am J Clin Nutr* **59**(3 Suppl): 747S–752S.

Miyashita, Y., N. Koide et al. (2004). "Beneficial effect of low carbohydrate in low calorie diets on visceral fat reduction in type 2 diabetic patients with obesity." *Diabetes Res Clin Pract* **65**(3): 235–241.

Montonen, J., D. Drogan et al. (2011). "Estimation of the contribution of biomarkers of different metabolic pathways to risk of type 2 diabetes." *Eur J Epidemiol* **26**(1): 29–38.

Mosdol, A., D. R. Witte et al. (2007). "Dietary glycemic index and glycemic load are associated with high-density-lipoprotein cholesterol at baseline but not with increased risk of diabetes in the Whitehall II study." *Am J Clin Nutr* **86**(4): 988–994.

Mozaffarian, D., T. Hao et al. (2011). "Changes in diet and lifestyle and long-term weight gain in women and men." *N Engl J Med* **364**(25): 2392–2404.

Mukherjee, S., G. Thakur et al. (2009). "Long-term effects of a carbohydrate-rich diet on fasting blood sugar, lipid profile, and serum insulin values in rural Bengalis." *J Diabetes* **1**(4): 288–295.

Murphy, M. M., J. S. Douglass et al. (2008). "Resistant starch intakes in the United States." *J Am Diet Assoc* **108**(1): 67–78.

Neyrinck, A. M., S. Possemiers et al. (2011). "Prebiotic effects of wheat arabinoxylan related to the increase in bifidobacteria, Roseburia and Bacteroides/Prevotella in diet-induced obese mice." *PLoS One* **6**(6): e20944.

Nimptsch, K., S. Kenfield et al. (2011). "Dietary glycemic index, glycemic load, insulin index, fiber and whole-grain intake in relation to risk of prostate cancer." *Cancer Causes Control* **22**(1): 51–61.

Nordmann, A. J., A. Nordmann et al. (2006). "Effects of low-carbohydrate vs low-fat diets on weight loss and cardiovascular risk factors: A meta-analysis of randomized controlled trials." *Arch Intern Med* **166**(3): 285–293.

Nuttall, F. Q., A. D. Mooradian et al. (1984). "Effect of protein ingestion on the glucose and insulin response to a standardized oral glucose load." *Diabetes Care* **7**(5): 465–470.

Odegaard, A. O., A. C. Choh et al. (2012). "Sugar-sweetened and diet beverages in relation to visceral adipose tissue." *Obesity (Silver Spring)* **20**(3): 689–691.

Odegaard, A. O., W. P. Koh et al. (2010). "Soft drink and juice consumption and risk of physician-diagnosed incident type 2 diabetes: The Singapore Chinese Health Study." *Am J Epidemiol* **171**(6): 701–708.

Palmer, J. R., D. A. Boggs et al. (2008). "Sugar-sweetened beverages and incidence of type 2 diabetes mellitus in African American women." *Arch Intern Med* **168**(14): 1487–1492.

Paolisso, G. and M. Barbagallo (1997). "Hypertension, diabetes mellitus, and insulin resistance: The role of intracellular magnesium." *Am J Hypertens* **10**(3): 346–355.

Paul, G. L., J. T. Rokusek et al. (1996). "Preexercise meal composition alters plasma large neutral amino acid responses during exercise and recovery." *Am J Clin Nutr* **64**(5): 778–786.

Pereira, M. A. (2006). "Weighing in on glycemic index and body weight." *Am J Clin Nutr* **84**(4): 677–679.

Pereira, M. A., D. R. Jacobs, Jr. et al. (2002). "Effect of whole grains on insulin sensitivity in overweight hyperinsulinemic adults." *Am J Clin Nutr* **75**(5): 848–855.

Pereira, M. A. and D. S. Ludwig (2001). "Dietary fiber and body-weight regulation. Observations and mechanisms." *Pediatr Clin North Am* **48**(4): 969–980.

Pereira, M. A., J. Swain et al. (2004). "Effects of a low-glycemic load diet on resting energy expenditure and heart disease risk factors during weight loss." *Jama* **292**(20): 2482–2490.

Pittler, M. H. and E. Ernst (2001). "Guar gum for body weight reduction: Meta-analysis of randomized trials." *Am J Med* **110**(9): 724–730.

Popkin, B. M. (2010). "Patterns of beverage use across the lifecycle." *Physiol Behav* **100**(1): 4–9.

Priebe, M. G., J. J. van Binsbergen et al. (2008). "Whole grain foods for the prevention of type 2 diabetes mellitus." *Cochrane Database Syst Rev*(1): CD006061.

Qi, L., J. B. Meigs et al. (2006). "Dietary fibers and glycemic load, obesity, and plasma adiponectin levels in women with type 2 diabetes." *Diabetes Care* **29**(7): 1501–1505.

Qi, L., E. Rimm et al. (2005). "Dietary glycemic index, glycemic load, cereal fiber, and plasma adiponectin concentration in diabetic men." *Diabetes Care* **28**(5): 1022–1028.

Qi, L., R. M. van Dam et al. (2006). "Whole-grain, bran, and cereal fiber intakes and markers of systemic inflammation in diabetic women." *Diabetes Care* **29**(2): 207–211.

Raben, A., T. H. Vasilaras et al. (2002). "Sucrose compared with artificial sweeteners: Different effects on ad libitum food intake and body weight after 10 wk of supplementation in overweight subjects." *Am J Clin Nutr* **76**(4): 721–729.

Riserus, U., W. C. Willett et al. (2009). "Dietary fats and prevention of type 2 diabetes." *Prog Lipid Res* **48**(1): 44–51.

Roberts, S. B. (2000). "High-glycemic index foods, hunger, and obesity: Is there a connection?" *Nutr Rev* **58**(6): 163–169.

Sacks, F. M., G. A. Bray et al. (2009). "Comparison of weight-loss diets with different compositions of fat, protein, and carbohydrates." *N Engl J Med* **360**(9): 859–873.

Sahyoun, N. R., A. L. Anderson et al. (2008). "Dietary glycemic index and glycemic load and the risk of type 2 diabetes in older adults." *Am J Clin Nutr* **87**(1): 126–131.

Salmeron, J., A. Ascherio et al. (1997). "Dietary fiber, glycemic load, and risk of NIDDM in men." *Diabetes Care* **20**(4): 545–550.

Salmeron, J., J. E. Manson et al. (1997). "Dietary fiber, glycemic load, and risk of non-insulin-dependent diabetes mellitus in women." *Jama* **277**(6): 472–477.

Samuel, V. T., K. F. Petersen et al. (2010). "Lipid-induced insulin resistance: Unravelling the mechanism." *Lancet* **375**(9733): 2267–2277.

Schulze, M. B., K. Hoffmann et al. (2005). "Dietary pattern, inflammation, and incidence of type 2 diabetes in women." *Am J Clin Nutr* **82**(3): 675–684; quiz 714–675.

Schulze, M. B., J. E. Manson et al. (2004). "Sugar-sweetened beverages, weight gain, and incidence of type 2 diabetes in young and middle-aged women." *Jama* **292**(8): 927–934.

Schulze, M. B., M. Schulz et al. (2007). "Fiber and magnesium intake and incidence of type 2 diabetes: A prospective study and meta-analysis." *Arch Intern Med* **167**(9): 956–965.

Schulze, M. B., M. Schulz et al. (2008). "Carbohydrate intake and incidence of type 2 diabetes in the European Prospective Investigation into Cancer and Nutrition (EPIC)-Potsdam Study." *Br J Nutr* **99**(5): 1107–1116.

Shimotoyodome, A., J. Suzuki et al. (2010). "RS4-type resistant starch prevents high-fat diet-induced obesity via increased hepatic fatty acid oxidation and decreased postprandial GIP in C57BL/6J mice." *Am J Physiol Endocrinol Metab* **298**(3): E652–E662.

Sievenpiper, J. L., C. W. Kendall et al. (2009). "Effect of non-oil-seed pulses on glycaemic control: A systematic review and meta-analysis of randomised controlled experimental trials in people with and without diabetes." *Diabetologia* **52**(8): 1479–1495.

Slabber, M., H. C. Barnard et al. (1994). "Effects of a low-insulin-response, energy-restricted diet on weight loss and plasma insulin concentrations in hyperinsulinemic obese females." *Am J Clin Nutr* **60**(1): 48–53.

Slavin, J. L. (2008). "Position of the American Dietetic Association: Health implications of dietary fiber." *J Am Diet Assoc* **108**(10): 1716–1731.

Slavin, J. L., M. C. Martini et al. (1999). "Plausible mechanisms for the protectiveness of whole grains." *Am J Clin Nutr* **70**(3 Suppl): 459S–463S.

Sloth, B., I. Krog-Mikkelsen et al. (2004). "No difference in body weight decrease between a low-glycemic-index and a high-glycemic-index diet but reduced LDL cholesterol after 10-wk ad libitum intake of the low-glycemic-index diet." *Am J Clin Nutr* **80**(2): 337–347.

Sluijs, I., Y. T. van der Schouw et al. (2010). "Carbohydrate quantity and quality and risk of type 2 diabetes in the European Prospective Investigation into Cancer and Nutrition-Netherlands (EPIC-NL) study." *Am J Clin Nutr* **92**(4): 905–911.

Sluijs, I., Y. T. van der Schouw et al. (2011). "Carbohydrate quantity and quality and risk of type 2 diabetes in the European Prospective Investigation into Cancer and Nutrition-Netherlands (EPIC-NL) study." *Am J Clin Nutr* **92**(4): 905–911.

Song, Y., K. He et al. (2006). "Effects of oral magnesium supplementation on glycaemic control in Type 2 diabetes: A meta-analysis of randomized double-blind controlled trials." *Diabet Med* **23**(10): 1050–1056.

Sorensen, L. B., A. Raben et al. (2005). "Effect of sucrose on inflammatory markers in overweight humans." *Am J Clin Nutr* **82**(2): 421–427.

Spranger, J., A. Kroke et al. (2003). "Inflammatory cytokines and the risk to develop type 2 diabetes: Results of the prospective population-based European Prospective Investigation into Cancer and Nutrition (EPIC)-Potsdam Study." *Diabetes* **52**(3): 812–817.

Stanhope, K. L. and P. J. Havel (2009). "Fructose consumption: Considerations for future research on its effects on adipose distribution, lipid metabolism, and insulin sensitivity in humans." *J Nutr* **139**(6): 1236S–1241S.

Stanhope, K. L., J. M. Schwarz et al. (2009). "Consuming fructose-sweetened, not glucose-sweetened, beverages increases visceral adiposity and lipids and decreases insulin sensitivity in overweight/obese humans." *J Clin Invest* **119**(5): 1322–1334.

Stevens, J., K. Ahn et al. (2002). "Dietary fiber intake and glycemic index and incidence of diabetes in African-American and white adults: The ARIC study." *Diabetes Care* **25**(10): 1715–1721.

Sun, Q., D. Spiegelman et al. (2010). "White rice, brown rice, and risk of type 2 diabetes in US men and women." *Arch Intern Med* **170**(11): 961–969.

Teff, K. L., S. S. Elliott et al. (2004). "Dietary fructose reduces circulating insulin and leptin, attenuates postprandial suppression of ghrelin, and increases triglycerides in women." *J Clin Endocrinol Metab* **89**(6): 2963–2972.

Teff, K. L., J. Grudziak et al. (2009). "Endocrine and metabolic effects of consuming fructose- and glucose-sweetened beverages with meals in obese men and women: Influence of insulin resistance on plasma triglyceride responses." *J Clin Endocrinol Metab* **94**(5): 1562–1569.

Thomas, D. and E. J. Elliott (2009). "Low glycaemic index, or low glycaemic load, diets for diabetes mellitus." *Cochrane Database Syst Rev*(1): CD006296.

Thomas, D. E., E. J. Elliott et al. (2007). "Low glycaemic index or low glycaemic load diets for overweight and obesity." *Cochrane Database Syst Rev*(3): CD005105.

Thorne, M. J., L. U. Thompson et al. (1983). "Factors affecting starch digestibility and the glycemic response with special reference to legumes." *Am J Clin Nutr* **38**(3): 481–488.

Tighe, P., G. Duthie et al. (2010). "Effect of increased consumption of whole-grain foods on blood pressure and other cardiovascular risk markers in healthy middle-aged persons: A randomized controlled trial." *Am J Clin Nutr* **92**(4): 733–740.

Tordoff, M. G. and A. M. Alleva (1990). "Effect of drinking soda sweetened with aspartame or high-fructose corn syrup on food intake and body weight." *Am J Clin Nutr* **51**(6): 963–969.

Tsai, C. J., M. F. Leitzmann et al. (2005). "Glycemic load, glycemic index, and carbohydrate intake in relation to risk of cholecystectomy in women." *Gastroenterology* **129**(1): 105–112.

United States Department of Agriculture (2010). "Report of the Dietary Guidelines Advisory Committee on the Dietary Guidelines for Americans, 2010," D5–1 to D5–65.

Vartanian, L. R., M. B. Schwartz et al. (2007). "Effects of soft drink consumption on nutrition and health: A systematic review and meta-analysis." *Am J Public Health* **97**(4): 667–675.

Vaughan, D. A., B.-R. Lu et al. (2008). "The evolving story of rice evolution." *Plant Science* **174**(4): 394–408.

Vega-Lopez, S. and S. N. Mayol-Kreiser (2009). "Use of the glycemic index for weight loss and glycemic control: A review of recent evidence." *Curr Diab Rep* **9**(5): 379–388.

Venn, B. J. and J. I. Mann (2004). "Cereal grains, legumes and diabetes." *Eur J Clin Nutr* **58**(11): 1443–1461.

Villegas, R., S. Liu et al. (2007). "Prospective study of dietary carbohydrates, glycemic index, glycemic load, and incidence of type 2 diabetes mellitus in middle-aged Chinese women." *Arch Intern Med* **167**(21): 2310–2316.

Vlassara, H., W. Cai et al. (2002). "Inflammatory mediators are induced by dietary glycotoxins, a major risk factor for diabetic angiopathy." *Proc Natl Acad Sci U S A* **99**(24): 15596–15601.

Voet, D. and J. G. Voet (2011). *Biochemistry*. New York, John Wiley & Sons.

Voss, S., A. Kroke et al. (1998). "Is macronutrient composition of dietary intake data affected by underreporting? Results from the EPIC-Potsdam Study. European Prospective Investigation into Cancer and Nutrition." *Eur J Clin Nutr* **52**(2): 119–126.

Wannamethee, S. G., P. H. Whincup et al. (2009). "Associations between dietary fiber and inflammation, hepatic function, and risk of type 2 diabetes in older men: Potential mechanisms for the benefits of fiber on diabetes risk." *Diabetes Care* **32**(10): 1823–1825.

Weickert, M. O., M. Mohlig et al. (2006). "CereaWeickert, M. O. and A. F. Pfeiffer (2008). "Metabolic effects of dietary fiber consumption and prevention of diabetes." *J Nutr* **138**(3): 439–442.

Westerterp, K. R., S. A. Wilson et al. (1999). "Diet induced thermogenesis measured over 24h in a respiration chamber: Effect of diet composition." *Int J Obes Relat Metab Disord* **23**(3): 287–292.

Whitney, E. and S. R. Rolfes (2008). *Understanding Nutrition*. Belmont, Wadsworth.

Willett, W. (2001). *Eat Drink, and Be Healthy*, Free Press, New York.

Willett, W. C., G. R. Howe et al. (1997). "Adjustment for total energy intake in epidemiologic studies." *Am J Clin Nutr* **65**(4 Suppl): 1220S–1228S.

Williams, P. G., S. J. Grafenauer et al. (2008). "Cereal grains, legumes, and weight management: A comprehensive review of the scientific evidence." *Nutr Rev* 66(4): 171–182.

Wolever, T. M., A. L. Gibbs et al. (2008). "The Canadian Trial of Carbohydrates in Diabetes (CCD), a 1-y controlled trial of low-glycemic-index dietary carbohydrate in type 2 diabetes: No effect on glycated hemoglobin but reduction in C-reactive protein." *Am J Clin Nutr* 87(1): 114–125.

World Health Organization/Food and Agriculture Organization (1998). Carbohydrates in human nutrition. (FAO Food and Nutiriton paper no. 66). Rome.

chapter three

Dietary fatty acids in the etiology of type 2 diabetes

Andrew O. Odegaard, PhD
University of Minnesota

Contents

Dietary intake is a significant factor in both primordial and primary prevention of type 2 diabetes through many avenues of influence as summarized in this book—all major macronutrients have been linked in one way or another to the etiology and prevention of type 2 diabetes. The focus of this chapter, though, is on research examining dietary fatty acids (FA) with clinical biomarkers thought to be central to the pathogenesis of type 2 diabetes, as well as studies on type 2 diabetes as an outcome.

The importance of dietary fat is underscored by its role as an essential factor in numerous vital functions in humans (Calder, Dangour et al. 2010). The multiple classes of dietary fat have a ubiquitous presence across food groups as dietary fat is ingested as a major and minor constituent in animal meats, fish, poultry/eggs, dairy, nuts/seeds, grains, vegetables, fruits, and legumes/pulses, not to mention oils which are derived from numerous sources. Oils are unique contributors as a source of dietary fat in the diet as they are 100% fat in composition, used as both a vehicle for cooking and as additions to foods and dishes across dietary patterns and populations. There are three major dietary fatty acid classes that are defined by their chain lengths, number, and position of double bonds (and thus overall structure). Saturated fatty acids (SFA) have no double bonds and are solid at room temperature, monounsaturated fatty acids (MUFA) have one double bond, polyunsaturated fatty acids (PUFA) have two or more double bonds, and MUFA and PUFA, unlike SFA, are liquid at room temperature. Within these classes, oleic acid (MUFA), linoleic acid (PUFA), palmitic acid (SFA), and stearic acid (SFA) are the most abundant fatty acids in the diets of most human populations (Hodson, Skeaff et al. 2008).

Trans-fatty acids (TFA) comprise a hybrid fourth class of dietary fatty acids as they are generally both MUFA and PUFA in structural form, but with a *trans* configuration rather than *cis*, although naturally occurring TFA from ruminants may be in the *cis* form. TFAs come from two major sources—industrial production (partial hydrogenation) and from ruminant animals. Industrial TFAs are produced artificially by heating liquid vegetable oils in the presence of metal catalysts and hydrogen (Ascherio, Katan et al. 1999). The partial hydrogenation causes the carbon atoms to bond in a straight configuration and remain in a solid state at room temperature (Ascherio, Katan et al. 1999). TFAs are produced in large quantities industrially to harden margarine, to turn vegetable oils into shortening, to lengthen shelf life by replacing fatty acids that would oxidize more quickly, and to give a certain "mouth feel" or flavor to deep-fried foods or other processed foods with added fats (Ascherio, Katan et al. 1999). TFAs are primarily consumed in bakery products, fast and fried foods, packaged snacks, and margarines. The main TFA isomers from industrial sources, which make up approximately more than 90% of TFA consumption (Gebauer, Psota et al. 2007), include elaidic acid (C18:1Δ9*t*) and linolelaidic acid (C18:2-*t*9*t*12). The evidence for TFAs increasing risk of cardiovascular disease is so consistent between observational and metabolic/experimental studies that the FDA demanded TFA content be included on all food labels (Ascherio, Katan et al. 1999). The result has been a considerable reduction in TFAs in the food supply over the past decade.

All foods with dietary fats, no exceptions, are mixtures of SFA, MUFA, and PUFA in different proportions. Dietary fat from animal meats, dairy products, and eggs are generally higher in SFA relative to fats from plants and oils, which are more unsaturated. However, it is important to note that the amounts and ratios of SFA, MUFA, and PUFA vary widely across the many types of animal and plant foods depending on a range of geographic, environmental, agricultural, and processing scenarios. Fatty acids are thus rarely consumed in isolation. This heterogeneity in the fat composition of our foods, and the correlations among the specific fatty acids within foods and dishes, is a fundamental basis of measurement error and confounding in nutritional epidemiology. An apt example and case study of this point is the FA profile from animal meat. On average, animal meat is predominately unsaturated in nature, with 40%–50% of FA being MUFA, 10%–20% being PUFA, and 30%–50% being SFA (Schmid 2011). Oleic acid (C18:1 n-9) (MUFA) is the most common FA found in meat, and the individual SFA most prominent are myristic (C14:0), palmitic (C16:0), and stearic (C18:0), with palmitic as the most common, making up ¼–1/3 of SFA, and stearic typically 10%–20% (Schmid 2011). The percentages vary by species of animal and anatomical location within animals, as well as many other characteristics such as rearing, feed, and climate/geography.

The reason for highlighting the heterogeneous nature of dietary fat in foods and the overall diet is to emphasize the complexity and difficulty in both carrying out and interpreting the research examining dietary fat as an exposure. The broad contribution of dietary FA from many sources showcases them as a central player with many roles in the orchestra of a whole dietary pattern. Overall, as summarized elsewhere in the book (see Dietary Patterns, Chapter 6), understanding the plausible mechanisms and precise pathways related to dietary FA and type 2 diabetes etiology should incorporate the concept of food synergy. Despite this complexity, there is a base of literature providing plausible biological models for the role of individual dietary FA in the pathophysiology of type 2 diabetes.

The mechanism whereby FA may impact the etiology of type 2 diabetes in humans is unclear. As with most other dietary components, it is likely that the potential biological effects of dietary FA are pleiotropic in nature. One major pathway of investigation includes the impact of FA on insulin sensitivity. This pathway is particularly plausible because cell membranes are comprised of phospholipids, and thus the specific types of dietary FA consumed is known to alter the physicochemical properties of cell membranes as they are incorporated into the membrane phospholipids (Borkman, Storlien et al. 1993; Storlien, Baur et al. 1996). Simply put, the types and ratios of dietary FA will affect the composition and function of the cells in the body. The FA composition of cell membranes will affect cellular functions including membrane fluidity, ion permeability, insulin receptor/binding affinity, and glucose transport (Ginsberg, Brown et al. 1981).

An additional pathway through which dietary FA may affect the etiology of type 2 diabetes is through FA effects on gene expression and enzyme activity (Hamajima, Hirose et al. 2002). It is through this pathway, especially with the PUFA linoleic acid, that an anti-inflammatory effect may occur (Willett 2007; Petersson, Basu et al. 2008). There is also evidence that dietary FA, especially PUFA, may inhibit hepatic lipogenesis and stimulate hepatic FA oxidation, which may improve insulin sensitivity (Hamajima, Hirose et al. 2002). In Figure 3.1, this theoretical model is outlined. It is important to note that these pathways have support from cellular in vitro studies and from animal studies. The of true pathways in humans has not yet been established.

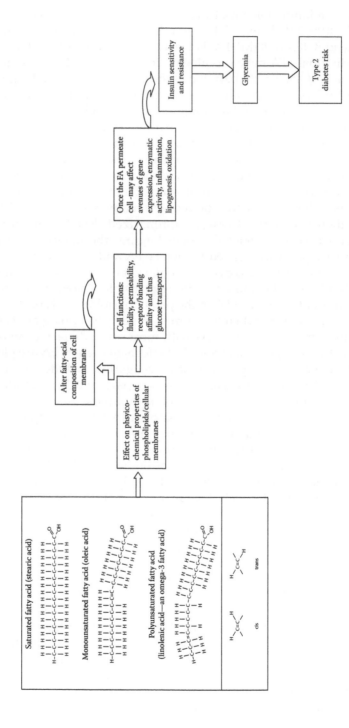

Figure 3.1 Theoretical mechanism whereby dietary fatty acids (FA) are involved in the etiology of type 2 diabetes.

Evidence Summary of Human and Population Based Research Related to Dietary Fatty Acids and Type 2 Diabetes								
	MUFA	PUFA (N-6)	PUFA (Marine N-3)	PUFA (Plant N-3)	N-6/N-3 Ratio	SFA	TFA (I)	TFA (R)
Evidence	⇔ ⇓	⇔ ⇓	⇐ ⇑⇑	⇔ ⇓	⇔	⇔ ⇑	⇑⇔	⇑⇑⇐

MUFA-Mono-unsaturated fatty acids
PUFA-Poly-unsaturated fatty acids
SFA-Saturated fatty acids
TFA-Trans-fatty acids (I = industrial, R = Ruminant)

⇑ = Increase in risk

⇓ = Decrease in risk

⇔ = Null

Figure 3.2 Evidence summary of human and population based research related to dietary fatty acids and type 2 diabetes.

Review of the literature

The following sections review and summarize the research salient to the role of dietary FA in etiology of type 2 diabetes. They are organized by study design due to the nature and intuition of research that has focused on substitution of one FA class for another. The human observational studies are focused on prospective studies with nondiabetics, as the goal here is to understand the role of dietary fat as a component of the diet in the cause and prevention of type 2 diabetes, rather than control of diabetes and secondary prevention. Study review sections are grouped according to randomized clinical trials of supplementation or feeding studies with biomarker endpoints relevant to the pathophysiology of type 2 diabetes, objectively measured biomarkers of FA intake with incident type 2 diabetes, and prospective observational studies with incident type 2 diabetes as the endpoint.

Randomized trials

A number of clinical trials have examined the effect of dietary FA with insulin sensitivity or another biomarkers and pathways relevant to the etiology of type 2 diabetes. One of the largest was a randomized parallel arm intervention trial in 162 nondiabetic men and women in Sweden, with a mean age of 49 years and mean BMI of 26.5 (Vessby, Unsitupa et al. 2001). The subjects were randomized to an isoenergetic diet (~37% total energy as fat) that contained either a high proportion of MUFA (21.2% E), or SFA (17.6% E) through dietary intake, and either a supplement pill of fish oil or placebo. This study was not a strict feeding study as participants received training, education, and guidance from dietitians on how to prepare and eat the specific diet. Dietary records were used to measure diet and adherence. The specific dietary composition data for each arm was not reported, but those on the SFA-enriched diet did consume less fiber, an important dietary marker and component related to insulin sensitivity. After 3 months, a frequently sampled intravenous glucose tolerance test was used to assess insulin sensitivity and secretion. Relative to the MUFA emphasized diet, the SFA diet resulted in significantly impaired insulin sensitivity, although there was no effect on glucose on either diet. There was no effect of the MUFA diet, so the overall results were due to a worsening of insulin resistance with greater SFA in the diet. The results were stronger in those who reported daily energy from dietary fat as <37% of total energy.

In another study testing a similar intake level of MUFA in 59 younger, healthy men and women (mean age 23, BMI 22.9 kg/m^2), participants went through a 3 period crossover trial (28 days each) with a base run-in diet high in SFA, compared to a MUFA-enriched diet, and a high-carbohydrate (CHO) diet. All diets were isocaloric. Relative to the SFA diet, the MUFA diet decreased fasting insulin, free fatty acids, and steady state plasma glucose. Overall, the MUFA diet improved insulin sensitivity relative to the SFA diet (Pérez-Jiménezk López-Miranda et al. 2011). Similar results were seen in a smaller study (n = 11) of older adults (mean age 62) who participated in a crossover study comparing higher fat diets either emphasizing SFA, CHO, or MUFA. Relative to SFA, MUFA improved Hba1c, fasting glucose, insulin, HOMA, and thus overall insulin sensitivity (Paniagua, de la Sacrista et al. 2007).

However, four different clinical trials found no effect of MUFA on any relevant measures relative to the etiology of type 2 diabetes. In a small study (n = 8) of healthy, lean men, provided four isocaloric diets in a crossover design, there was no effect of high MUFA on any parameters relevant to glucose/insulin metabolism (Fasching, Batheiser et al. 1996). It is possible the very short study time of 1 week per period, and compensatory metabolic capacity of the subjects precluded any generalization of the results. In a population similar to the aforementioned study, 15 healthy, lean young women were fed two isocaloric diets for 28 days, high in fat and emphasizing either MUFA or SFA, and found no effects of MUFA or SFA on any parameters of insulin or glucose (Louheranta, Turpeinen et al. 1998). A similar study also carried out a crossover trial where healthy young adults (n = 25) (mean age 28) were fed isocaloric diets enriched with MUFA or SFA and observed no significant effects on any insulin or glucose parameters (Lovejoy, Smith et al. 2002). Lastly, 18 moderately overweight, hyperlipidemic men (mean age 40) were fed 2 isocaloric diets for 3 weeks (Lithander, Keough et al. 2008). Each saw no effect of a MUFA + PUFA enriched diet versus a SFA diet on adiponectin, an insulin-sensitizing cytokine secreted from adipose tissue (Lithander, Keough et al. 2008). The only main methodological point for discussion from this study is the

little actual variation in the fat in the diets in addition to the limited duration. Overall, there was scant reporting of overall dietary characteristics in
the study groups across each study, limiting the interpretation of all these
studies.

The randomized studies are not limited to the above described trials. What follows are individual descriptions of studies directly or indirectly testing effects of different fatty acids and FA profiles on parameters
related to the etiology of type 2 diabetes. In a parallel arm trial including
417 men and women with metabolic syndrome, comparisons were made
between diets enriched with either MUFA or SFA, low fat with omega-3
FA, or low fat with no omega-3 FA, and the outcomes were markers of
oxidative stress or inflammation (Petersson, Basu et al. 2008). Participants
were randomized to 1 of the 4 diets for 12 weeks and received dietary
instruction and specific supplemental items to meet the dietary fatty acid
profiles and overall macronutrient profiles. Overall, there was no effect of
any of the diets on markers of oxidative stress or inflammation.

In 78, untreated hypertensive adults, a double blind-placebo controlled
trial compared fish oil supplementation versus corn oil at levels of 4 g/day
for 16 weeks (Deacon, Nauck et al. 1995). The participants were overweight
and generally healthy middle-aged adults. Compared to the corn oil placebo, there was no effect of N-3 fish oil supplementation on any parameters
of glucose metabolism in this population. An important consideration in
the interpretation of this study is that corn oil is not inert and is comprised
of mainly PUFA and MUFA with less SFA and a small amount of N-3 in
the form of alpha-linolenic acid as part of the overall PUFA.

A study of 15 healthy, normal-weight women participated in a randomized crossover feeding study comparing the effects of substituting
4% of energy from the SFAs, Lauric acid C12:0, and Palmitic C16:0 in place
of MUFA on glucose metabolism (Schwab, Niskanen et al. 1995). Over the
4 weeks of each of the periods, there were no effects of the different proportion of these SFA on glucose metabolism.

Sixty-three overweight women with abdominal obesity participated
in a randomized parallel arm trial comparing dietary supplementation
with industrial TFA, ruminant TFA, or neither (Tardy, Lambert-Porcheron
et al. 2009). Participants were given dietary guidance and products to
meet the desired FA profile for each arm. Compliance was assessed by
dietary records during the run in week and last week of the intervention,
and measurement of fatty acid plasma phospholipid profile, which was
shown to be correlated. Insulin sensitivity was assessed using a euglycemic clamp. After 4 weeks of emphasizing a dietary fat intake profile
aligning with these aims, there was no difference between any measure
of insulin sensitivity or glycemia between the arms.

Another randomized crossover feeding study of 28 day periods in
14 young, healthy, normal-weight women compared the effects of diets

with higher MUFA versus TFA substituted for SFA on glucose and lipid metabolism (Louheranta, Turpeinen et al. 1999). The TFA-enriched diet did not alter any parameters related to glycemia or insulin sensitivity compared to the MUFA-enriched diet, but as a proof of concept, did alter the lipid ratios unfavorably. In a similar trial of 31 participants, mean age 56, with obesity and impaired glucose tolerance, randomization to a diet emphasizing MUFA or PUFA while holding SFA constant for 8 weeks was carried out (Louheranta, Sarkkinen et al. 2002). This intervention followed an initial run in diet emphasizing SFA for 3 weeks. Participants received guidance and products to meet the dietary fatty acid profile aims for each arm. Both the MUFA and PUFA arms observed a decrease in fasting glucose relative to the SFA run in, but the MUFA arm was borderline significantly different than the PUFA at the $P < 0.05$ level. Oleic (MUFA) and ALA (N-3) were the FA with the most influence according to the change in serum phospholipid fatty acid composition of the participants, thus explaining a portion of the results. Similar to previous trials, overall dietary details and composition was not reported, and the use of fasting glucose as the endpoint, with its known vagaries, need to be considered in the interpretation. The different length of the comparison diet (SFA) is another consideration.

An extensive study of 36 overweight but generally healthy men and women, mean age 63, were randomized in a crossover feeding study of six 35-day periods. The periods emphasized a different experimental fat and thus fatty acid profile (Lichtenstein, Erkkilä et al. 2003). Overall, the periods emphasizing shortening, and thus TFA and butter (SFA), both displayed significantly higher levels glucose, insulin, and HOMA relative to the other dietary fats. A similar study participant profile that included 15 men and women, mean age 64, who were overweight and generally healthy, also completed a 4 period (35 days each), randomized crossover feeding study that emphasized different oils and thus fatty acid profiles (Vega-López, Ausman et al. 2006). The hydrogenated oil (TFA)-enriched diet had the greatest HOMA and insulin values, followed by the Palm (SFA) diet, both of these values were significantly greater than the soybean and canola (PUFA and MUFA), respectively. There were no significant differences in glucose. These results suggest that TFA and SFA as part of overall and common oils negatively influence insulin sensitivity relative to oils emphasizing MUFA and PUFA in content.

Lefevre and colleagues (2005) conducted an experimental investigation of the single-meal acute effects of C18:1 *cis* versus *trans* FA on postprandial glycemia, insulinemia, and lipemia. Twenty-two moderately overweight men and women were fed a basal 24% fat diet for 16 days. On days 10 and 16, they were fed a large (40% of daily energy needs) high-fat (50% of energy) meal in a randomized crossover design. This meal included 15% of energy as C18:1 *cis* fatty acid on one day, while on the other day 10% of the C18:1 *cis* was replaced with C18:1 *trans*. From this study, the absolute amount of C18:1 *trans* that was fed to the subjects is unclear. Nonetheless, the results support the hypothesis that replacing *cis* with *trans* may acutely exacerbate insulin resistance after only a single high-fat meal, as indicated by high-postprandial insulinemia and C-peptide concentrations following the *trans* treatment (Lefevre, Lovejoy et al. 2005). The last study reviewed addressing TFA (*trans* fatty acids), with a randomized component, reports the results of a dietary intervention in 52 overweight, but otherwise healthy postmenopausal women who were randomized to receive either partially hydrogenated soybean oil (15 g/d TFA) or a control oil (mainly oleic and palmitic acid) for 16 weeks (Bendsen, Stender et al. 2011). Results showed that the controlled dietary intervention did not significantly alter insulin sensitivity, β-cell function, or the metabolic clearance rate of insulin; also unchanged was the ability of insulin to suppress plasma nonesterified fatty acids and glycerol during oral glucose ingestion.

Griffin, Sanders et al. (2006) tested an n-6/n-3 ratio of 3:1/5:1 compared to a ratio of 10:1 in a parallel arm dietary intervention of men and women aged of 45–70 years in the United Kingdom in general good health. Insulin sensitivity was the outcome; however, no evidence was found of any effects of the lower ratio or overall omega-3 fatty acid intake on any measures of insulin sensitivity. The study intervention was based on foods, rather than on supplements, and a fairly rigid design was imposed on other parameters. The greater majority of participants (60%) were insulin resistant, and a larger proportion were taking medications (Griffin, Sanders et al. 2006). Minihane et al. also examined the question in a population susceptible to diabetes, and found no effect of a high n-6/n-3 ratio on insulin sensitivity or any related (Minihane, Brady et al. 2005).

Riserus, Arner et al. (2002) examined the effect of 1% of energy from *trans*-10, *cis*-12 conjugated linoleic acid (CLA) on insulin sensitivity in abdominally obese men with risk factors for the metabolic syndrome, and found significantly decreased insulin sensitivity compared to a placebo (Riserus, Arner et al. 2002). A similar study by Riserus, Vessby et al. (2004) using the same design and a similar population tested the effect of 1% of energy from *cis*-9, *trans*-11 against a placebo, and found that this isomer of CLA also induced a significant decline in insulin sensitivity. A 50:50 mix of the two isomers did not produce any statistically significant results compared to the placebo intake (Risérus, Vessby 2004).

Overall summary of the randomized trials

Overall, half of the studies examining SFA show no effect of high SFA intake on short- to mid-term levels of measures related to glycemia/insulin sensitivity compared to unsaturated FA, whereas the other half show worsening levels for diabetes risk based on the measured factors. Of the studies examining industrial (hydrogenated) TFA, two demonstrated worsened insulin sensitivity/glycemia measures and four were null. No effect of ruminant and a suggestive negative effect of CLA were observed. Of interest, MUFA and PUFA did not necessarily improve measures of insulin sensitivity or glycemia in any study. Thus, they essentially only had null effects, but in comparison to SFA or TFA in a mix of studies they had positive effects. On the other hand, SFA and TFA also did not improve any measures of insulin sensitivity or glycemia. In short, if there was movement in any of the biomarkers in any of the periods or arms of these studies, it occurred with higher levels of SFA and TFA and resulted in worsened levels of insulin sensitivity and glycemia. What would seem to be essential to a critical appraisal of these studies is the lack of any summary or detailed reporting of overall dietary characteristics. As well, very few of the studies reported on any physical activity levels during the study or other factors that could influence the measures of interest.

Studies of objectively measured FA intake and incident type 2 diabetes mellitus (T2DM)

The ARIC study prospectively investigated the relation of plasma cholesterol ester (CE) and phospholipid (PL) fatty acid composition with the incidence of diabetes mellitus (Wang, Folsom et al. 2003). The study included 2909 adults aged 45–64 years; plasma fatty acid composition was quantified by gas–liquid chromatography and was expressed as a percentage of total fatty acids. Incident diabetes ($n = 252$) was identified during 9 years of follow-up. Plasma PL and CE reflects dietary intake weeks to months before the collection of the sample. Collectively, MUFA were not associated with CE measures and suggestively inversely associated with PL measures. Plasma MUFAs did not reflect dietary MUFAs ($r \leq 0.05$), as would be expected given their endogenous synthesis. The proportional saturated fatty acid composition of plasma was positively associated with the development of diabetes. For N-6 PUFA, CE, and PL measures, there was an inverse relationship between greater linoleic acid composition and incident type 2 diabetes, whereas overall levels of PUFA were not associated. For N-3 PUFA, PL measures displayed an inverse relationship between greater alpha-linolenic acid (ALA) composition and incident type 2 diabetes, and no association with CE measures. Overall, levels of n-3 PUFA were not associated with type 2 diabetes. An important point for this study and others is that the measurement of tissue fatty acid composition does not perfectly represent the proportion of fatty acids in the diet because of variability between individuals in the cellular utilization and endogenous synthesis of fatty acids (Wang, Folsom et al. 2003).

Also, individual fatty acids were expressed as proportions of total fatty acids. Because endogenously synthesized fatty acids are included in the denominator, and the total fatty acid proportions must sum to 100%, proportional fatty acid measurements are inherently interdependent, both biologically and mathematically. That is, a high percentage of SFAs will automatically reflect a low percentage of unsaturated fatty acids. This makes it difficult to interpret the effect of single fatty acid constituents independent of other fatty acids.

A nested case-cohort study within EPIC investigated erythrocyte membrane FA levels, desaturase activity, and self-reported dietary FA in relation to the incidence of type 2 diabetes (Huuskonen, Vaisanen et al. 2000). Desaturases are enzymes that catalyze the synthesis and conversion of different fatty acids. This study included 2724 participants (673 incident cases). Overall, there was no association between total MUFA, PUFA, SFA, or TFA measured in the erythrocyte membrane and risk of diabetes. Similar to the prior reviewed study, erythrocyte FA were expressed as the percentages of total FA, and dietary FA were expressed as a percentage of total fat intake. Thus, it was difficult to interpret results for individual FA independent of the other FA.

In 1,828 50-year-old men, the fatty acid composition in serum cholesterol esters was assessed in the years 1970–1973 in Finland and followed up 10 years on average (Vessby, Aro et al. 1994). The results demonstrated that the 75 men who developed diabetes had significantly higher proportions of the saturated fatty acids with 14 (myristic acid) and 16 (palmitic acid) carbon atoms, a higher proportion of palmitoleic acid (16:1w-7), and a considerably lower proportion of linolenic acid (18:2w-6). They also had higher proportions of [gamma]-linolenic (18:3w-6) and dihomo-[gamma]-linolenic (20:3w-6) acids in serum, but there were no differences with respect to the N-3 fatty acids. The main dietary sources of myristic acid (14:0), palmitic acid (16:0), and palmitoleic acid (16:1w-7) are different types of meat and dairy products, but as noted, these fatty acids are also synthesized by the body.

In 895 men in the Kuopio Ischemic Heart Disease Risk Factor study, mean age 53, who had serum fatty acid composition measured, 56 developed impaired fasting glucose and 34 developed type 2 diabetes over 4 years of follow-up (Laaksonen, Lakka et al. 2002). The authors concluded there was no association with MUFA, as the measures likely represent as the synthesis from SFA or endogenous production more so than intake. They also observed that men with greater PUFA (linoleic acid) serum fatty acid measurements had a more stable glycemic profile and lesser risk of developing IFG or type 2 diabetes.

In 3,088 men and women, mean age 75 in the Cardiovascular Health Study, plasma phospholipid N-3 FA were measured and incident diabetes was determined over a median of 10.6 years of follow-up (Djoussé et al. 2011).

This objective measure approximates intake over the previous 3 weeks. With increasing marine-based plasma phospholipid N-3 FA (EPA + DHA), there was a suggestive inverse association with developing type 2 diabetes, and with increasing plant-based N-3 (alpha-linolenic Acid, ALA), there was a strong inverse association. Similar results were observed with ALA in data derived from an FFQ, but the results were null with marine-based N-3.

In 3,737 adults from the Melbourne Cohort Study with plasma phospholipid data on fatty acid%, the investigators carried out a prospective case-cohort study on incident diabetes (Hodge, English et al. 2007). Participants were men and women, approximate mean age 55, and were followed 4 years after baseline measurement. The authors found no association between MUFA or PUFA plasma phospholipid levels and type 2 diabetes, a positive association between SFA and diabetes, and a strong inverse association between TFA plasma phospholipid levels and diabetes. Of note, related to the TFA results were the very low levels and narrow distribution that suggests a questionable representation of TFA.

In the EPIC-Norfolk nested case–control study examining incident diabetes, including 199 incident cases and 184 controls, plasma phospholipid and erythrocyte-membrane fatty acid fractions were measured (Patel, Sharp et al. 2010). Participants were on average 64 years of age at baseline and differed strongly by BMI level. The results were generally inconsistent between the two objective methods, with only some general consistency of a positive association with a greater level of SFA according to either measure. Overall, there was no association with MUFA, an inverse association with plasma for PUFA, a positive association with plasma with SFA, and no association with TFA.

A unique endeavor using the Cardiovascular Health Study population examined an exogenous source of the dietary fatty acid—*trans*-palmitoleate, which is primarily found naturally in dairy and other ruminant trans fats, and does not show an increased risk of CVD (Micha, Wallace et al. 2010). This study examined the association between plasma phospholipid *trans*-palmitoleate and incident type 2 diabetes. Plasma-phospholipid represents midterm intake in duration of fatty acids. Although intake of this fatty acid is a minor part of the diet, the data observed support the role of this and other certain fatty acids (e.g., n-3) having a powerful role on physiologic function related to glucose/insulin metabolism. Increased measures of this fatty acid, which correlate strongly with whole and low fat dairy foods and red meat intake, were strongly associated with lower fasting insulin levels, insulin resistance, triglycerides. As well, a strong, inverse dose–response association with incident type 2 diabetes was observed, with adjustment for numerous lifestyle and dietary factors not materially affecting the results. Because the levels of this fatty acid are so low, it is appropriate to raise the question of whether they are truly an active compound given the very small range of this FA, or a marker of some other unknown constituent, possibly of dairy or ruminants foods.

Summary of the studies with objective measures of fatty acids

Overall, these studies observed essentially no association between measured MUFA and type 2 diabetes, about half that measured PUFA, including N-3, showed an inverse association with higher measured levels, and the majority but not all of the studies examining SFA levels displayed a positive association, with TFA displaying a range of effects from positive to inverse, with qualifications. There was also varying associations between the naturally occurring TFA in dairy and meat from ruminants relative to industrial TFA. A strength of these studies is that the majority were able to thoroughly account for potential confounders. The objective measures are also a strength, but the aforementioned points on what they actually represent are vital for interpretation since the length of intake is variable, the objective measures also represent endogenous production, and the relative proportions of intake merit careful and cautious interpretation. Similar to the randomized trials with biomarkers related to glucose and insulin metabolism, there were no strong congruencies between the studies on specific FA. Overall, similar to the randomized studies, these studies of objectively measured fatty acids suggest that if SFA and TFA have any effect on the etiology of type 2 diabetes it is likely negative (i.e., increased risk), whereas if there is any effect of MUFA or PUFA it is likely positive (i.e., decreased risk). However, more consistent findings in with strongly designed studies will be needed to draw clear inferences from this body of literature.

Prospective observational studies with self-reported dietary intake

The Nurses' Health Study examined dietary FA intake in estimates derived from a repeated and validated FFQ in 84,204 women, mean age 46 years and followed for 14 years (Salmeron, Hu et al. 2001). Diabetes incidence was assessed and validated in the cohort. Statistical modeling has important implications for the epidemiologic investigation of dietary fatty acids since there tends to be significant correlations between the different classes of fatty acids, and with total energy. In the current study, nutrient density modeling was performed to account for statistical issues related to this sort of study design (Willett 1998). The results from the study were null for MUFA and SFA intake, with a strong inverse association with overall PUFA, and a strong positive association with greater TFA intake. For marine N-3 fatty acids, the RRs for increasing quintiles of fatty acids were 1.0 (reference), 1.00 (95% CI: 0.88, 1.13), 0.93 (0.81, 1.06), 0.97 (0.84, 1.12), and 0.80 (0.67, 0.95); the *P* for the trend was 0.02. Similar results were observed with a substitution modeling approach.

In an analysis from the Iowa Women's Health Study that included 35,988 postmenopausal women aged 55–69 free of diabetes and without extreme reported caloric intake (Meyer, Kushi et al. 2001). The diabetes outcome was self-reported over 11 years of follow-up and 1,890 women reported developing type 2 diabetes. A validation study of the report of diabetes was conducted on 85 participants, 44 who reported yes and 41 who reported no. There was perfect specificity of the report, but only 28 of the 44 who reported developing type 2 diabetes had a confirmatory report from their physician, suggesting there may be overreporting of diabetes in this population. Dietary intake was assessed at baseline in 1986 with the 127 item Willett FFQ, and validated with 24 h recalls. The authors used the residual method in their analysis for energy adjustment of the individual fatty acids. No association was observed between dietary MUFA, SFA, TFA, and N-3 with incident diabetes, but a significant inverse association between PUFA intake and type 2 diabetes risk was observed.

In the Health Professionals Follow-up Study including 42,504 men who were free of major chronic disease and without extreme reported dietary intakes at baseline in 1986, an analysis of dietary fat and type 2 diabetes risk was carried out (van Dam, Willett et al. 2002). Dietary intake was assessed with a 131-item FFQ 3 times (1986, 1990, 1994), a particular strength of the study. Participants were followed through 1998. Diabetes was self-reported and further confirmed with a supplemental questionnaire on symptoms, diagnostic tests, and medications, and showed a high level of validity. The analysis appeared to be carried out appropriately using energy density and residual methods depending on the fatty acid. The results showed no association between MUFA, SFA, TFA, marine N-3, and nonmarine N-3 FA with type 2 diabetes risk. The results for PUFA were also null, but in a subgroup analysis of men < 65 years of age and BMI < 25 kg/m², there was an inverse association between *N*-6 linoleic acid and incident diabetes.

The EPIC Norfolk study examined diabetes incidence in relation to dietary fat intake in 23,631 Caucasian men and women aged 40–78 in the years 1993–1998 and followed up for 3–7 years (Harding, Day et al. 2004). The study aimed to examine the pattern of dietary fat intake by looking at the polyunsaturated to saturated fat ratio (P:S) based on self-reported habitual dietary data from a 127-item FFQ similar to that used in the Nurses' Health Study. The FFQ was validated using weighed food records in a subsample of participants and had similar correlation coefficients for validity to other large observational prospective studies of diet and chronic disease. Type 2 diabetes was self-reported and then verified through registries, hospital admissions, medical records, and death certificates. After the validation efforts, it appeared there were both under- and overreporting of the development of diabetes, and the cases considered were formally valid. These efforts likely represent a conservative number of cases based on the nature of the disease. Participants were free of major chronic disease and did not report unusual dietary intake at baseline to be included. Statistical methods appropriated dietary fat as percent of total energy in the analysis (density). The final model included the ratio, total fat as a percentage of total energy, protein (% energy), total energy, and alcohol. The results indicated an inverse association with increasing P:S ratio until adjustment for adiposity. While adjustment for total fat, protein, and energy did not affect the estimate, it is important to consider what this model represents in actual interpretation given the exposure is a ratio of two fatty acids.

In the observational follow-up of participants in the Women's Health Study, 36,328 women, mean age 54.6 were followed from 1992–2008 for incident type 2 diabetes and 2370 cases were identified (Djoussé, Gaziano et al. 2011). The Women's Health Study was developed as a randomized, double-blind placebo-controlled trial to study the effects of low-dose aspirin and Vitamin E on primary prevention of cardiovascular disease and cancer in 1992–2004. Women were excluded in this analysis if they had prevalent or unclear diabetes status at baseline, or nonnormal or missing reported dietary intake. Diabetes status was self-reported and validated by either phone interview or supplemental questionnaire utilizing American Diabetes Association criteria. Positive-predictive value of the diabetes outcome was reported at 91%. Dietary intake was assessed using a 128 item FFQ and was validated. The study aimed to examine omega-3 FA intake with incident type 2 diabetes. Marine (EPA, DHA, DPA) FA were derived from reported intake from the FFQ and an increased risk with increasing levels of overall marine N-3, as well as its major components (EPA, DHA) was observed in a dose-dependent manner across quintiles of intake as follows: relative risk = 1.0 (referent), 1.17 (95% confidence interval: 1.03, 1.33), 1.20 (1.05, 1.38), 1.46 (1.28, 1.66), and 1.44 (1.25, 1.65), respectively (P for trend = 0.0001). Interpretation of these findings needs to consider the statistical models used to derive them. This study adjusted for all other fatty acids except MUFA; and also included red meat as a covariate, which is a major contributor to SFA, MUFA, and PUFA in the diet. Furthermore, meat is a food rather than a nutrient. There was no specific adjustment for overall protein or carbohydrate intake as a portion of the diet, whereas both fiber and glycemic index were included in the model. Thus, the model employed does not approach the question it is meant to answer in a fashion consistent with traditional nutritional epidemiological approaches aiming to examine this question (Willett 1998). The adjustment for meat and both GI and fiber may also represent overadjustment. One last point to consider in interpretation of the results from this study is the narrow range of N-3 FA derived from the FFQ data. Specifically, the range of mean or median values for quintile of EPA were 0.01, 0.02, 0.03, 0.08, 0.12 g/day, and this was associated with a stepwise increase in the fully adjusted model (hazard ratios = 1.00, 1.08, 1.25, 1.30, 1.38, P < 0.0001). Thus, the data suggest that even with a very low intake and range there is a powerful stepwise association with increased intake. Similar associations were observed for DHA intake ranging from 0.04, 0.09, 0.12, 0.17, 0.17 g/day in each quintile. Because the levels of these fatty acids are so low, it is appropriate to raise the question of whether they are truly the active causal agent given the very small range of the FA, or a marker of some other unknown constituent or confounder.

A study of a Dutch population aimed to investigate the relation between eicosapentaenoic acid (EPA) and docosahexaenoic acid (DHA) intake and risk of type 2 diabetes in a population-based cohort of 4,472 men and women age 55 and above (mean age ~68), free of diabetes, and without unusual dietary intake (van Woudenbergh, van Woudenbergh et al. 2009). Participants enrolled from 1990–1993 and were followed through 2005. A 170-item FFQ was used to assess usual dietary intake at baseline. Levels of EPA and DHA, as well as other nutrients were derived from the data. Diabetes was assessed by monitoring general practitioner and pharmacy databases. Overall, there was no association between EPA and DHA levels as derived from the FFQ and incidence of type 2 diabetes. The statistical models that produced the results did not adjust for physical activity as most participants did not have these data available, and there was also minimal adjustment for other dietary confounders (TFA, fiber, selenium, vitamin D, total energy). Data were not presented with any adjustment for body habitus as well. And no report was given on the study of validity of the FFQ in the population.

In a study of over 195,000 men and women from the Nurses' Health Study and Health Professional's Study, investigators examined marine N-3 and nonmarine N-3 (ALA) with incidence of type 2 diabetes updating previous analyses and providing more in depth analysis (Kaushik, Mozaffarian et al. 2009). All participants were free of major chronic disease and had usual defined dietary intakes at baseline assessment with validated FFQ, with repeated assessment. Diabetes was self-reported and validated. The analyses examined nutrient intake using the residual method. Data from the HPS displayed no association between intake of N-3 FA and developing diabetes, whereas in the NHS increased intake of N-3 was positively associated with incident type 2 diabetes. Intakes between the two studies were pooled and examined individually showing inconsistent results, as they depended on the grouping (quintiles versus deciles) and were driven by the NHS. ALA was also examined, but the results appeared to be null.

In an investigation of 43,176 middle-aged and older (ages 45–74 at baseline in 1993–98) Chinese men and women living in Singapore who were free of major chronic disease and without extreme report of dietary intake, the association between PUFA and incident type 2 diabetes was examined (Brostow, Odegaard et al. 2011). Dietary intake was assessed using a 165-item FFQ specifically developed and validated within the study population along with a specific nutrient composition database, and type 2 diabetes was assessed by self-report then validated using hospital discharge databases, a telephone interview inquiring on symptoms, tests, and therapies, plus HbA1c measures in a random subsample. Overall, very strong validity was observed for those reporting incident diabetes, and there was evidence from the HbA1c that approximately 5% of participants who did not report diabetes had levels of HbA1c higher than levels considered diabetic. Thus, there was potential underreporting of cases, a widely accepted point related to the natural history and clinical diagnosis of type 2 diabetes. The residual method was used for the fatty acids in the statistical analysis, and the approach was complete. There was no association between levels of N-6 PUFA as derived from the reported dietary intake and incident type 2 diabetes. There was also no association between MUFA and incident type 2 diabetes. For total N-3 FA intake from both marine and nonmarine sources, there was a stepwise inverse association with increasing intake. However, upon parsing the source of the N-3 FA, it was clear this association was driven by nonmarine sources (ALA), as a strong inverse association was observed between ALA and type 2 diabetes risk. On the other hand, there was no association between marine-based N-3 and incident type 2 diabetes. A novel contribution in this study was the examination of the N-6:N-3 FA ratio. This ratio has been hypothesized as being important in relation to chronic disease (Simopoulos 2008); however, there is little evidence to support this claim, and this study of Chinese men and women was also null in this respect.

In the Shanghai Men's and Women's Health Studies, 51,963 men and 64,193 women free of major chronic disease were included in analyses examining N-3 intake derived from FFQ data (Villegas, Xiang et al. 2011). Participants did not report extreme dietary intakes, and the FFQ was validated. The women's study commenced in 1996 and participants were followed through 2006, and the men's study initiated in 2002 and participants were followed through 2008. Type 2 diabetes was self-reported in both studies, and was confirmed if the case status met American Diabetes Association criteria. Statistical models relating N-3 intake in quintiles with incident diabetes were adjusted for BMI, waist–hip ratio, lifestyle and demographic factors, and overall dietary pattern scores as derived from the complete FFQ data. The adjustment for overall dietary pattern slightly attenuated the estimates. Overall, the median levels of marine N-3 by quintile of intake were low (0.02, 0.04, 0.07, 0.11, 0.20 g/day). In the women's study, an inverse association with greater levels of N-3 intake was observed, but in the men's study, there was no association. The analytic approach in this study was unique relative to the other published prospective studies on dietary fatty acids as the overall dietary pattern was included as a covariate. However, this adjustment appeared to have had little effect on the point estimates. Another consideration in the interpretation is the short follow-up time in men, on average about 4 years. Lastly, similar to other studies, the overall range of N-3 intake is within a low and narrow range, so aforementioned caveats of interpretation on what this may actually represent apply.

Summary of findings from observational prospective studies

The overall summary results from the observational prospective studies with incident type 2 diabetes differ in subtle ways from studies under the other design umbrellas. First, both MUFA and SFA were null across studies and populations. Similar to the other study groups, N-6 PUFA displayed inverse associations in some studies but was null in others. Overall, N-3 FA from marine sources exhibited inverse associations in some studies, positive in others, as well as being null in some. On the other hand, nonmarine sources of N-3 (ALA) were either inverse or null in their associations with type 2 diabetes. There was a range of methodological approaches applied in the studies and statistical models, which could contribute to the equivocal nature of the findings. It is also possible, due to the diverse nature of the populations examined, that these individual fatty acid levels actually represent different sources and overall dietary patterns. Indeed, there is a high probability that much of the true nature of dietary fats and disease risk is "lost in translation" over the course of extracting data from these studies and statistically analyzing them with complicated models. People do not eat FA in isolation; they eat them in combinations within and across foods and dishes, a subject covered in Chapter 6.

The body of research that examines dietary fat intake in the etiology of type 2 diabetes highlights the complexity and difficulty of studying the topic. To date, there is no wholly conclusive data on any individual FA in respect to diabetes risk. Although the overall data are equivocal in nature precluding any firm conclusions on the individual role of different fatty acid classes, there were some minor consistent trends within the different classes. The association between MUFA and markers for diabetes risk or actual type 2 diabetes was generally null, although a few studies displayed a possible beneficial relationship relative to SFA or TFA. The results relating to N-6 PUFA were very similar in nature, either displaying no relationship or potential benefit with greater levels in the diet. N-3 PUFA displayed greater variance with some studies showing a beneficial role, some null, and some suggesting an increased risk. This was especially the case with marine-based N-3 FA, but less so with nonmarine N-3 (ALA), as this plant-based FA was either null or protective of risk, but also less studied. Findings on the overall N-6 to N-3 ratio suggested no association with risk of type 2 diabetes.

Research on SFA and type 2 diabetes risk, or diabetes risk factors, demonstrated either null associations or potentially an increased risk with higher SFA intake. Research on TFA was similar, with some evidence suggesting a harmful role, some null, and some even suggestive of protective associations. Despite the lack of clarity for TFA in relation to diabetes risk, the accepted role of TFA in increasing the risk for cardiovascular disease should take precedence in dietary recommendations. Studies of FA consumed in very small quantities originating from ruminant animals also display a range of associations from protective to harmful, and this specific issue is worthy of further studies that may bring clarity to the question.

In sum, the inconsistent results across FA classes with type 2 diabetes underlines the need to continue to carefully study the topic, update related study methods, analytical approaches, and creatively examine the subject matter. They also stress the need to interpret any results in the spectrum of the overall dietary pattern, so the fatty acid intake has some context. Dietary fat plays an essential and critical role in human biological function; however, the role of different FA classes in the etiology and prevention of type 2 diabetes has some general direction but remains inconclusive.

References

Ascherio, A., Katan, M. B., Zock, P. L., Stampfer, M. J., and Willett, W. C. (1999). "Trans fatty acids and coronary heart disease." *N Engl J Med* **340**(25): 1994–1998.

Bendsen, N. T., Stender, S., Szecsi, P. B., Pedersen, S. B., Basu, S., Hellgren, L. I., Newman, J. W., Larsen, T. M., Haugaard, S. B., and Astrup, A. (2011). "Effect of industrially produced trans fat on markers of systemic inflammation: Evidence from a randomized trial in women." *J Lipid Res* **52**(10): 1821–1828.

Borkman, M., Storlien, L. H., Pan, D. A. et al. (1993). "The relation between insulin sensitivity and the fatty-acid composition of skeletal muscle phospholipids." *N Engl J Med* **328**: (238–244).

Brostow, D. P., Odegaard, A. O. et al. (2011). "Omega-3 fatty acids and incident type 2 diabetes: The Singapore Chinese Health Study." *Am J Clin Nutr* **94**(2): 520–526.

Calder, P. C., Dangour, A. D., Diekman, C., Eilander, A., Koletzko, B., Meijer, G. W., Mozaffarian, D., Niinikoski, H., Osendarp, S. J., Pietinen, P., Schuit, J., and Uauy, R. (2010). "Essential fats for future health. *Proceedings of the 9th Unilever Nutrition Symposium*, May 26–27, 2010." *Eur J Clin Nutr* **64**(suppl. 4): S1–13.

Deacon, C. F., Nauck, M. A. et al. (1995). "Both subcutaneously and intravenously administered glucagon-like peptide I are rapidly degraded from the NH2-terminus in type II diabetic patients and in healthy subjects." *Diabetes* **44**(9): 1126–1131.

Djoussé, L., Biggs, M. L., Lemaitre, R. N., King, I. B., Song, X., Ix, J. H., Mukamal, K. J., Siscovick, D. S., and Mozaffarian, D. (2011). "Plasma omega-3 fatty acids and incident diabetes in older adults." *Am J Clin Nutr* **94**(2): 527–533.

Djoussé, L., Gaziano, J. M., Buring, J. E., and Lee, I. M. (2011). "Dietary omega-3 fatty acids and fish consumption and risk of type 2 diabetes." *Am J Clin Nutr* **93**(1): 143–150.

Fasching, P., Ratheiser, K., Schneeweiss, B., Rohac, M., Nowotny, P., and Waldhäusl, W. (1996). "No effect of short-term dietary supplementation of saturated and poly- and monounsaturated fatty acids on insulin secretion and sensitivity in healthy men." *Ann Nutr Metab* **40**(2): 116–122.

Gebauer, S., Psota, T. L., Kris-Etherton, P. M. (2007). "The diversity of health effects of individual trans fatty acid isomers." *Lipids* **42**: 787–799.

Ginsberg, B. H., Brown, T. J., Simon, I., Spector, A. A. (1981). "Effect of the membrane lipid environment on the properties of insulin receptors." *Diabetes* **30**(9): 773–780.

Griffin, M., Sanders, T. A. B., Davies, I. G. et al. (2006). "Effects of altering the ratio of n-6 to n-3 fatty acids on insulin sensitivity, lipoprotein size, and postprandial lipemia in men and postmenopausal women aged 45–70 y: The OPTILIP study." *Am J Clin Nutr* **84**: 1290–1298.

Hamajima, N., Hirose, K. et al. (2002). "Alcohol, tobacco and breast cancer—collaborative reanalysis of individual data from 53 epidemiological studies, including 58,515 women with breast cancer and 95,067 women without the disease." *Br J Cancer* **87**(11): 1234–1245.

Harding, A. H., Day, N. E., Khaw, K. T., Bingham, S., Luben, R., Welsh, A., and Wareham, N. J. (2004). "Dietary fat and the risk of clinical type 2 diabetes: The European prospective investigation of Cancer-Norfolk study." *Am J Epidemiol* **159**(1): 73–82.

Hodge, A. M., English, D. R., O'Dea, K., and Giles, G. G. (2007). "Dietary patterns and diabetes incidence in the melbourne collaborative cohort study." *Am J Epidemiol* **165**(6): 603–610.

Hodson, L., Skeaff, C. M., and Fielding, B. A. (2008). "Fatty acid composition of adipose tissue and blood in humans and its use as a biomarker of dietary intake." *Prog Lipid Res* **47**(5): 348–380.

Huuskonen, J., Vaisanen, S. B. et al. (2000). "Determinants of bone mineral density in middle aged men: A population-based study." *Osteoporos Int* **11**(8): 702–708.

Kaushik, M., Mozaffarian, D., Spiegelman, D., Manson, J. E., Willett, W. C., and Hu, F. B. (2009). "Long-chain omega-3 fatty acids, fish intake, and the risk of type 2 diabetes mellitus." *Am J Clin Nutr* **90**(3): 613–620.

Laaksonen, D. E., Lakka, T. A., Lakka, H. M., Nyyssönen, K., Rissanen, T., Niskanen, L. K., Salonen, J. T. (2002). "Serum fatty acid composition predicts development of impaired fasting glycaemia and diabetes in middle-aged men." *Diabet Med* **19**(6): 456–464.

Lefevre, M., Lovejoy, J. C. et al. (2005). "Comparison of the acute response to meals enriched with cis- or trans-fatty acids on glucose and lipids in overweight individuals with differing FABP2 genotypes." *Metabolism* **54**(12): 1652–1658.

Lichtenstein, A. H., Erkkilä, A. T., Lamarche, B., Schwab, U. S., Jalbert, S. M., and Ausman, L. M. (2003). "Influence of hydrogenated fat and butter on CVD risk factors: Remnant-like particles, glucose and insulin, blood pressure and C-reactive protein." *Atherosclerosis* **171**(1): 97–107.

Lithander, F. E., Keogh, G. F., Wang, Y., Cooper, G. J., Mulvey, T. B., Chan, Y. K., McArdle, B. H., and Poppitt, S. D. (2008). "No evidence of an effect of alterations in dietary fatty acids on fasting adiponectin over 3 weeks." *Obesity* **16**(3): 592–599.

Louheranta, A. M., Sarkkinen, E. S., Vidgren, H. M., Schwab, U. S., and Uusitupa, M. I. (2002). "Association of the fatty acid profile of serum lipids with glucose and insulin metabolism during 2 fat-modified diets in subjects with impaired glucose tolerance." *Am J Clin Nutr* **76**(2): 331–337.

Louheranta, A. M., Turpeinen, A. K. et al. (1999). "A high-trans fatty acid diet and insulin sensitivity in young healthy women." *Metabolism* **48**(7): 870–875.

Louheranta, A. M., Turpeinen, A. K., Schwab, U. S., Vidgren, H. M., Parviainen, M. T., and Uusitupa, M. I. (1998). "A high-stearic acid diet does not impair glucose tolerance and insulin sensitivity in healthy women." *Metabolism* **47**(5): 529–534.

Lovejoy, J. C., Smith, S. R., Champagne, C. M., Most, M. M., Lefevre, M., DeLany, J. P., Denkins, Y. M., Rood, J. C., Veldhuis, J., and Bray, G. A. (2002). "Effects of diets enriched in saturated (palmitic), monounsaturated (oleic), or trans (elaidic) fatty acids on insulin sensitivity and substrate oxidation in healthy adults." *Diabetes Care* **25**(8): 1283–1288.

Meyer, K. A., Kushi, L. H., Jacobs, D. R. Jr., and Folsom, A. R. (2001). "Dietary fat and incidence of type 2 diabetes in older Iowa women." *Diabetes Care* **24**(9): 1528–1535.

Micha, R., Wallace, S. K., and Mozaffarian, D. (2010). "Red and processed meat consumption and risk of incident coronary heart disease, stroke, and diabetes mellitus: A systematic review and meta-analysis." *Circulation* **121**(21): 2271–2283.

Minihane, A., Brady, L. M., Lovegrove, S. S. et al. (2005). "Lack of effect of dietary n-6:n-3 PUFA ratio on plasma lipids and markers of insulin responses in Indian Asians living in the UK." *Eur J Nutr* **44**(1): 26–32.

Paniagua, J. A., de la Sacristana, A. G., Sánchez, E., Romero, I., Vidal-Puig, A., Berral, F. J., Escribano, A., Moyano, M. J., Peréz-Martinez, P., López-Miranda, J., and Pérez-Jiménez, F. (2007). "A MUFA-rich diet improves posprandial glucose, lipid and GLP-1 responses in insulin-resistant subjects." *J Am Coll Nutr* **26**(5): 434–444.

Patel, P. S., Sharp, S. J., Jansen, E., Luben, R. N., Khaw, K. T., Wareham, N. J., and Forouhi, N. G. (2010). "Fatty acids measured in plasma and erythrocyte-membrane phospholipids and derived by food-frequency questionnaire and the risk of new-onset type 2 diabetes: A pilot study in the European Prospective Investigation into Cancer and Nutrition (EPIC)-Norfolk cohort." *Am J Clin Nutr* **92**(5): 1214–1222.

Pérez-Jiménez, F., López-Miranda, J., Pinillos, M. D., Gómez, P., Paz-Rojas, E., Montilla, P., Marín, C., Velasco, M. J., Blanco-Molina, A., Jiménez Perepérez, J. A., and Ordovás, J. M. (2011). "A Mediterranean and a high-carbohydrate diet improve glucose metabolism in healthy young persons." *Diabetologia* **44**(11): 2038–2043.

Petersson, H., Basu, S., Cederholm, T., and Risérus, U. (2008). "Serum fatty acid composition and indices of stearoyl-CoA desaturase activity are associated with systemic inflammation: Longitudinal analyses in middle-aged men." *Br J Nutr* **99**(6): 1186–1189.

Riserus, U., Arner, P., Brismar, K. et al. (2002). "Treatment with dietary trans10cis12 conjugated linoleic acid causes isomer-specific insulin resistance in obese men with the metabolic syndrome." *Diabetes Care* **25**: 1516–1521.

Risérus, U., Vessby, B., Arnlöv, J., and Basu, S. (2004). "Effects of cis-9, trans-11 conjugated linoleic acid supplementation on insulin sensitivity, lipid peroxidation, and proinflammatory markers in obese men." *Am J Clin Nutr* **80**(2): 279–283.

Salmeron, J., Hu, F. B. et al. (2001). "Dietary fat intake and risk of type 2 diabetes in women." *Am J Clin Nutr* **73**(6): 1019–1026.

Schmid, A. (2011). "The role of meat fat in the human diet." *Crit Rev Food Sci Nutr* **51**(1): 50–66.

Schwab, U. S., Niskanen, L. K., Maliranta, H. M., Savolainen, M. J., Kesäniemi, Y. A., Uusitupa, M. I. (1995). "Lauric and palmitic acid-enriched diets have minimal impact on serum lipid and lipoprotein concentrations and glucose metabolism in healthy young women." *J Nutr* **125**(3): 466–473.

Simopoulos, A. P. (2008). "The importance of the omega-6/omega-3 fatty acid ratio in cardiovascular disease and other chronic diseases." *Exp Biol Med* **233**(6): 674–688.

Storlien, L. H., Baur, L. A. et al. (1996). "Dietary fats and insulin action." *Diabetologia* **39**(6): 621–631.

Tardy, A. L., Lambert-Porcheron, S., Malpuech-Brugère, C., Giraudet, C., Rigaudière, J. P., Laillet, B., Leruyet, P., Peyraud, J. L., Boirie, Y., Laville, M., Michalski, M. C., Chardigny, J. M., Morio, B. (2009). "Dairy and industrial sources of trans fat do not impair peripheral insulin sensitivity in overweight women." *Am J Clin Nutr* **90**(1): 88–94.

van Dam, R. M., Willett, W. C., Rimm, E. B., Stampfer, M. J., and Hu, F. B. (2002). "Dietary fat and meat intake in relation to risk of type 2 diabetes in men." *Diabetes Care* **25**(3): 417–424.

van Woudenbergh, G. J., van Ballegooijen, A. J., Kuijsten, A., Sijbrands, E. J., van Rooij, F. J., Geleijnse, J. M., Hofman, A., Witteman, J. C., and Feskens, E. J. (2009). "Eating fish and risk of type 2 diabetes: A population-based, prospective follow-up study." *Diabetes Care* **32**(11): 2021–2026.

Vega-López, S., Ausman, L. M., Jalbert, S. M., Erkkilä, A. T., and Lichtenstein, A. H. (2006). "Palm and partially hydrogenated soybean oils adversely alter lipoprotein profiles compared with soybean and canola oils in moderately hyperlipidemic subjects." *Am J Clin Nutr* **84**(1): 54–62.

Vessby, B., Aro, A., Skarfors, E. et al. (1994). "The risk to develop NIDDM is related to the fatty acid composition of the serum cholesterol esters." *Diabetes* **43**(1353–1357).

Vessby, B., Unsitupa, M., Hermansen, K. et al. (2001). "Substituting dietary saturated for monounsaturated fat impairs insulin sensitivity in healthy men and women: The KANWU Study." *Diabetologia* **44**: 312–319.

Villegas, R., Xiang, Y. B., Elasy, T., Li, H. L., Yang, G., Cai, H., Ye, F., Gao, Y. T., Shyr, Y., Zheng, W., and Shu, X. O. (2011). "Fish, shellfish, and long-chain n-3 fatty acid consumption and risk of incident type 2 diabetes in middle-aged Chinese men and women." *Am J Clin Nutr* **94**(2): 543–551.

Wang, L., Folsom, A. R., Zheng, Z. J., Pankow, J. S., Eckfeldt, J. H., ARIC Study Investigators (2003). "Plasma fatty acid composition and incidence of diabetes in middle-aged adults: The Atherosclerosis Risk in Community.

Willett, W. C. (1998). *Nutritional Epidemiology*. New York, Oxford University Press.

Willett, W. C. (2007). "The role of dietary n-6 fatty acids in the prevention of cardiovascular disease." *J Cardiovasc Med (Hagerstown)*(suppl.): s42–45.

chapter four

Proteins, amino acids, and type 2 diabetes

Yan Song, MD, MS and Simon Liu, MD, ScD

Contents

Introduction

Diet plays an important role in affecting type 2 diabetes risk. Recently, interest in dietary protein intake has increased in diabetes research, resulting in an emerging body of human and animal studies linking protein intake to glucose metabolism, insulin sensitivity, and risk of type 2 diabetes. This chapter provides a summary of these studies assessing the roles of dietary proteins in the development of type 2 diabetes. We first review relevant biochemical functions and metabolism as well as food sources of protein and amino acids. We then review the previous studies on the relation between dietary proteins and amino acid intake and type 2 diabetes in human populations.

Proteins and amino acids

Proteins

Protein is the most abundant organic compound in cells. Excluding water, protein accounts for about half of body weight and plays critically important structural and functional roles in humans. There are various functional roles of proteins in humans, as follows:

1. As enzymes, proteins act as biological catalysts that facilitate biochemical reactions in the body. For instance, *hexokinase* phosphorylates a hexose to its active version—a hexose phosphate; *pepsin* degrades food proteins into peptides; *DNA polymerase* catalyzes the polymerization of deoxyribonucleotides into a DNA strand. Enzymes facilitate biochemical reactions without being changed in the process.
2. As hormones, some proteins directly regulate biologic processes. In response to glucose stimulation, for example, insulin is a polypeptide released by the pancreas and promotes the utilization of glucose by peripheral tissues.
3. As transporters, some proteins such as *hemoglobin* can transport oxygen and carbon dioxide in red blood cells. *Sex hormone binding globulin* (SHBG) binds testosterone and estradiol in bloodstream sequestering sex steroids from their biological functions.
4. As building blocks, proteins form the basic structure of nearly all organs in the body. Spleens, lungs, and muscles have the highest content of protein (more than 80% dry weight), whereas bones and teeth have the lowest. Even in the low-protein-content tissues as bones and teeth, to build their structure, the body needs a matrix of *collagen* (a type of protein) and then fills it with crystals of different minerals (such as calcium, phosphorus, and magnesium). Structural proteins in living bodies are constantly replaced.
5. As antibodies, some proteins such as *immunoglobulin can* combat the invasion of intruders such as bacteria and viruses. Also, *thrombin* and *fibrinogen* participate in the procedure of coagulation, thus preventing the body from excessive hemorrhage.

6. As a source of energy and glucose, proteins can be sacrificed to provide energy through biological oxidation, as well as to produce glucose through gluconeogenesis.
7. There are also other roles of proteins. For example, *actin* and *myosin* cause the contraction of skeletal muscles, which form the basis of all human movement; *keratin*, which is tough and insoluble, is the key structural material making up the outer layer of skin, hair, and nails.

Amino acids

The basic building blocks of proteins are amino acids. All amino acids have the same basic structure (Figure 4.1) including a central α-carbon (C), a hydrogen (H), an amino group (-NH$_2$), and a carboxylic acid group (-COOH), along with a side group (-R) that serves to distinguish different amino acids (20 different amino acids listed in Table 4.1).

There are nine amino acids that the human body cannot produce endogenously, or cannot produce sufficiently to meet its needs. These amino acids are called *essential amino acids* (Table 4.1). These must come from dietary intake. The other 11 amino acids that can be produced endogenously are not necessarily needed from external food sources. Generally, the more essential amino acids a certain protein contains, the higher nutrition value it has.

Each amino acid is connected to the next one by a peptide bond (Figure 4.2). The polypeptide chain is the structural basis for proteins. Most proteins are dozens to hundreds or thousands amino acids long. The sequence of amino acid residues of a protein is called its *primary structure*. For example, the primary structure of human insulin A chain is "N-C-Y-N-E-L-Q-Y-L-S-C-V-S-A-C-C-Q-E-V-I-G." Depending on its primary structure, the polypeptide chain twists into certain complex and tangled shapes. The local spatial substructures that are highly regular are called the *secondary structure* of a protein. Two main types of secondary structure of proteins are the α-helix and β-sheet. *Tertiary structure* of

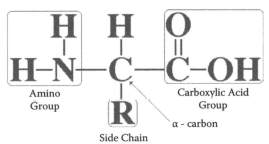

Figure 4.1 Basic structure of amino acids.

Table 4.1 Amino Acids that Are Most Common in Proteins

Essential amino acids			Nonessential amino acids		
Name	3-Letter acronym	Single-letter acronym	Name	3-Letter acronym	Single-letter acronym
Valine	Val	V	Arginine	Arg	R
Isoleucine	Ile	I	Alanine	Ala	A
Leucine	Leu	L	Proline	Pro	P
Threonine	Thr	T	Serine	Ser	S
Methionine	Met	M	Tyrosine	Tyr	Y
Lysine	Lys	K	Glutamine	Gln	Q
Phenylalanine	Phe	F	Asparagine	Asn	N
Tryptophan	Trp	W	Cysteine	Cys	C
Histidine	His	H	Glycine	Gly	G
			Aspartic acid	Asp	D
			Glutamic acid	Glu	E

a protein refers to its three-dimensional structure in which the α-helixes and β-sheets are folded into a compact globule together. Some proteins (e.g., hemoglobin) comprise several polypeptide chains. The relative spatial relation of the subunits in a protein is called its *quaternary structure* (see Table 4.2.).

Digestion and absorption of protein

Only if the proteins are digested into amino acids and small peptides, they can be absorbed and utilized by the organism. The enzyme that digests proteins in the stomach is *pepsin*. Pepsin cleaves proteins into smaller fragments—small peptides and some amino acids. The hydrochloric acid in the stomach helps to disentangle the spatial structure of proteins to

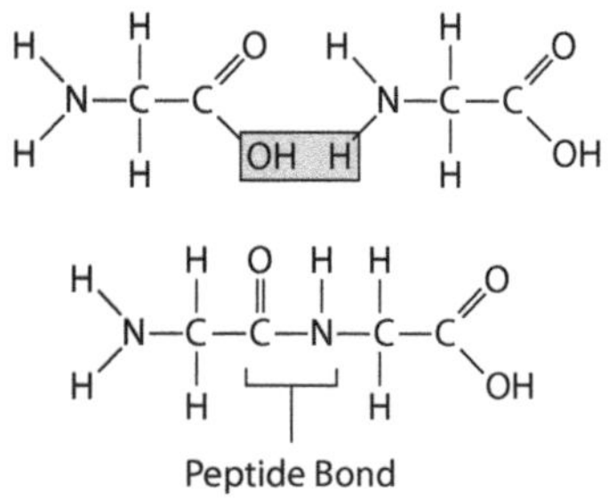

Peptide Bond

Figure 4.2 Peptide bond formulated by two molecules of glycine.

Table 4.2 Molecular Information for Selected Proteins of Humans

Protein	Number of amino acid residues	Number of polypeptide chains
Cytochrome C	104	1
Hemoglobin	574	4
Albumin	~550	1
Immunoglobulin G (IgG)	~1320	4
Apolipoprotein B (Apo B)	4636	1

facilitate its digestion (the most suitable pH for pepsin to work is 1.5~2.5). After entering the small intestine, polypeptides are further digested by proteases and peptidases into mostly single amino acids. The major organ that generates proteases is the pancreas. The pancreatic proteases include *trypsin, chymotrypsin, elastase, carboxypeptidase,* and *collagenase,* whereas *oligopeptidase* is generated by the small intestine. It is estimated that about 95% of the dietary proteins can be digested thoroughly (Mahe, Marteau et al. 1994; Evenepoel, Claus et al. 1999).

Protein absorption occurs (single amino acids, some dipeptides, and tripeptides) in the small intestine. Different specific carriers that transport these products are located in the membranes of small intestine cells. These carriers transport amino acids into the intestinal cells. This process is an ATP-consuming active transportation process. Once getting into the intestinal cells, the amino acids are either used in these cells or transported outside the cells into the surrounding fluid where they enter the circulation.

Metabolism of amino acids

Exogenous amino acids derived from dietary proteins form the amino acid metabolic pool together with endogenous amino acids generated from either the breakdown of tissue protein or synthesized by other sources. Under different metabolic conditions, amino acids in the metabolic pool lose their amino groups to form α-ketoacids, which is the carbon skeleton of amino acids. The α-ketoacids undergo different metabolic pathways: either converted into glucose by gluconeogenesis, or degraded into CO_2 and H_2O by oxidation. The amino groups that were also generated from the metabolism of amino acids are converted into urea through the *ornithine cycle,* which is an important detoxification process of amines. Figure 4.3 shows the process of amino acid metabolism in the human body.

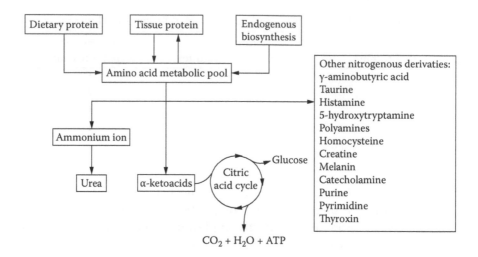

Figure 4.3 The catabolism process of amino acids.

Proteins in foods

There are two essential properties in evaluating proteins in foods: quantity and quality. The *quantity* of protein is how much protein a certain food contains per unit weight or serving. The *quality* of protein refers to the amino acids composition and their relative proportion in certain food. Generally, animal sources of proteins, including meat, dairy product, egg, poultry, and fish, are considered good quality. They contain a balanced level of amino acids that is most suitable for humans, and are readily digested and absorbed. For plant proteins, legumes (soy products, peas, beans, etc.) are most similar to animal proteins. The limiting amino acids in certain food determine its nutritional value. Proteins from vegetable sources tend to be deficient in one or more essential amino acids. For example, legumes are deficient in methionine and tryptophan but contain a large amount of isoleucine and lysine.

Dietary proteins and type 2 diabetes

Dietary proteins play important roles in modulating glucose metabolism and insulin sensitivity (Tremblay, Lavigne et al. 2007). Under isocaloric conditions, higher intake of protein will lead to lower intake of other macronutrients, namely, fat and carbohydrate. In short-term studies (≤6 months), dietary protein intake lowers the intake of calories at the expense of carbohydrates, which could improve glycemic control (Promintzer and Krebs 2006). In long-term studies (>1 year, see

Table 4.3 for details), however, numerous studies in different populations indicated that dietary protein from animal sources, but not from
plant sources was associated with a higher risk of type 2 diabetes after
a follow-up period of 4–10 years (relative risk on the scale of 1.21–2.15)
(Sluijs, Beulens et al. 2010).

Proteins and body weight

High-protein low-carbohydrate diets (usually with ≥30% total energy provided by protein) are often recommended by nutritionists or bodybuild-
ers to help to build muscle and lose fat. Two kinds of high-protein diets
are well known. The *Atkins diet* was created by Robert Atkins (Atkins
2001), which emphasizes the restriction of carbohydrate and consumption of proteins ad libitum. The *Montignac diet* was invented by Michel
Montignac (Montignac 2003), which focuses on reducing the intake of
high glycemic index carbohydrates and increasing the intake of proteins.

High-protein diets may enhance body weight loss, compared to conventional total energy restriction diets (Hu 2005). Previous randomized
trials consistently showed that "high-protein diets" (with ~30% total
energy provided by protein) resulted in greater weight loss than "stan-
dard-protein diets" (with ~15% total energy provided by protein) (see
Table 4.4). High-protein diets also were shown to increase lean mass and
decrease blood lipid concentrations (Samaha, Iqbal et al. 2003; McAuley,
Hopkins et al. 2005; McAuley, Smith et al. 2006; Soenen and Westerterp-
Plantenga 2010).

Two potential mechanisms are proposed to explain the effect of
high-protein diets in weight control. One is that the intake of proteins
can promote satiety signals to reduce the further consumption of calories
(Weigle, Breen et al. 2005). Some studies showed that high-protein diets
could decrease the level of circulating *ghrelin*, an orexigenic gut peptide,
and could increase the concentrations of anorexic peptides such as *chole-
cystokinin, glucagon-like peptide* 1, and *peptide YY* (Batterham, Heffron et al.
2006; Blom, Lluch et al. 2006; Tannous dit El Khoury, Obeid et al. 2006).
The other potential mechanism is that high-protein diets may increase
energy expenditure, which results in negative energy balance. The thermic response to a protein meal was largest and most prolonged, compared with a carbohydrate meal and a fat meal (Nair, Halliday et al. 1983).
Uncoupling proteins (UCP) are also thought to be mediating the protein-
induced energy expenditure increase. Studies have shown that high-protein diets could increase UCP2 in the liver and UCP1 in brown adipose
tissue. The increase of UCP levels was associated with higher energy
expenditure (Petzke, Riese et al. 2007). Thus, dietary protein intake could
affect type 2 diabetes through its influence on body weight.

Table 4.3 Population Study Evidence of the Association between Dietary
Protein Intake and Type 2 Diabetes Risk

Reference	Follow-up time (years)	Study type	Population	Adjustment	Effect size
De Koning et al. 2011 (deKoning, Fung et al. 2011)	20	Cohort	HPFS, 40,475 male health professionals	Age, smoking, physical activity, coffee intake, alcohol intake, family history of T2D, total energy intake, and body mass index	High animal protein and fat: 1.37 (1.20–1.58) High vegetable protein and fat: 0.95 (0.84–1.07)
Wang et al. 2010 (Wang, deKoning et al. 2010)	—	Cross-sectional	146 South Asian Indians aged 45–79 years	Age, sex, waist circumference, and hypertension	Total protein:1.70 (1.08–2.68) per SD
Sluijs et al. 2010 (Sluijs, Beulens et al. 2010)	10	Cohort	38,094 participants of the European Prospective Investigation into Cancer and Nutrition (EPIC)-NL study	Unadjusted	Total protein: 2.15 (1.77–2.60) Animal protein: 2.18 (1.80–2.63) Vegetable protein: 0.84 (0.70–1.01)

Table 4.3 Population Study Evidence of the Association between Dietary
Protein Intake and Type 2 Diabetes Risk (continued)

Reference	Follow-up time (years)	Study type	Population	Adjustment	Effect size
Villegas et al. 2008 (Villegas, Gao et al. 2008)	4.6	Cohort	64,227 middle-aged Chinese women	Age, energy intake, BMI, waist-to-hip ratio, smoking, alcohol consumption, vegetable intake, fiber, physical activity, income level, education level, occupation, and hypertension	Soy protein: 0.88 (0.75–1.04)
Wolever et al. 1997 (Wolever, Hamad et al. 1997)	—	Cross-sectional	728 residents from Ontario > 9 years	Age, sex, and BMI	Total protein: 1.38 (1.04–1.83) per SD
Duc Son le et al. 2005 (Duc Son le, Hanh et al. 2005)	—	Case-control	144 adult Vietnamese subjects	Family history of diabetes, socioeconomic status, smoking habit, and energy intake	Total protein: 1.21 (1.12–1.31) Animal protein: 1.18 (1.10–1.26)

Table 4.4 Studies on the Relation between Dietary Intake of Protein and Obesity or Body Weight

Reference	Follow-up time	Study type	Population	Adjustment	Effect size
Bujnowski et al. 2011 (Bujnowski, Xun et al. 2011)	7 years	Cohort	1,730 employed white men aged 40 to 55	Age, education, cigarette smoking, alcohol intake, energy, carbohydrate and saturated fat intake, and history of diabetes or other chronic disease	Animal protein: 4.62 (2.68–7.98) Vegetable protein: 0.58 (0.36–0.95)
Joo et al. 2011 (Joo, Park et al. 2011)	12 weeks	Nonrandomized trial	515 overweight adult Korean subjects	Unadjusted	BMI decrease: −1.9 ± 0.1 (high-protein diet) versus −1.1 ± 0.3 (conventional diet) (P < 0.05)
Soenen et al. 2010 (Soenen and Westerterp-Plantenga 2010)	3 months	RCT	24 adults	Unadjusted	Fat mass: −0.6 ± 0.8 kg (high-protein diet) versus 0.1 ± 0.5 kg (control) (P < 0.05) Lean mass increase: 0.9 ± 0.6 (high-protein diet) versus 0.2 ± 0.7 kg
McAuley et al. 2005 (McAuley, Hopkins et al. 2005)	24 weeks	RCT	96 normoglycemic, insulin-resistant women, BMI > 27	Baseline variables that were varied across the three groups	Greater reduction of body weight, waist circumference, and triglycerides in the Atkins diet and Zone diet groups than in the high-carbohydrate, high-fiber diet

Reference	Duration	Design	Subjects	Adjustment	Results
McAuley et al. 2006 (McAuley, Smith et al. 2006)	12 months	RCT	93 overweight insulin-resistant women	Baseline variables	Substantial sustained improvement in waist circumference, triglycerides and insulin in the Zone diet group than in the high-carbohydrate, high-fiber diet and Atkins diet group
Foster et al. 2003 (Foster, Wyatt et al. 2003)	1 year	RCT	63 obese men and women	Unadjusted	The low-carbohydrate high-protein high-fat diet group lost more weight than the conventional group (low-calorie high-carbohydrate low-fat): 3 months −6.8 ± 5.0 versus −2.7 ± 3.7% body weight; 6 months −7.0 ± 6.5 versus −3.2 ± 5.6; 12 months −4.4 ± 6.7 versus −2.5 ± 6.3
Samaha et al. 2003 (Samaha, Iqbal et al. 2003)	6 months	RCT	132 severely obese subjects	Unadjusted	Low-carbohydrate diet (with significantly higher intake of protein) lost more weight than the low-fat diet group: −5.8 ± 8.6 kg versus −1.9 ± 4.2 kg Greater decreases in triglyceride: −20 ± 43% versus −4 ± 31%

(continued)

Table 4.4 Studies on the Relation between Dietary Intake of Protein and Obesity or Body Weight (continued)

Reference	Follow-up time	Study type	Population	Adjustment	Effect size
Stern et al. 2004 (Stern, Iqbal et al. 2004)	1 year	RCT	132 obese adults	Age, race, sex, baseline body mass index, baseline caloric intake, and the presence or absence of hypertension, lipid-lowering therapy use, diabetes, active smoking, and sleep apnea	Greater weight loss in the low-carbohydrate diet (with significantly higher intake of protein) than in the low-fat diet group: −5.1 ± 8.7 kg versus −3.1 ± 8.4 kg Greater decrease in triglyceride: −0.65 ± 1.78 versus 0.05 ± 0.96 mmol/L Less decrease in HDL cholesterol: −0.03 ± 0.18 versus −0.13 ± 0.16 mmol/L
Brinkworth et al. 2004 (Brinkworth, Noakes et al. 2004)	52 weeks	RCT	58 obese, nondietetic subjects with hyper-insulinemia	Unadjusted	Greater weight loss in high-protein (30%) diet than in standard protein (15%) diet: −4.1 ± 5.8% versus −2.9 ± 3.6% (nonsignificant)

Study	Duration	Design	Subjects	Analysis	Outcome
Sargrad et al. 2005 (Sargrad, Homko et al 2005)	8 weeks	RCT	12 T2D patients	Unadjusted	Greater weight loss in high-protein (30%) diet group than in standard protein (15%) group (nonsignificant)
Lusconbe et al. 2002 (Luscombe, Clifton et al. 2002)	12 weeks	RCT	26 obese subjects with T2D	Unadjusted	Greater weight loss in high-protein (28%) diet group than in low-protein diet (16%) group (nonsignificant)

Effects on insulin secretion and function

Dietary proteins affect insulin secretion and action as well. The effects of protein intake on insulin and glucose metabolism differ between short-term and long-term intake. Short-term (days) dietary protein intake was shown to stimulate insulin secretion and reduce blood glucose concentration (Spiller, Jensen et al. 1987; Remer, Pietrzik et al. 1996) (see Table 4.5), whereas long-term (months or years) high-protein diets also increases insulin secretion, but decreases overall insulin sensitivity, and enhances gluconeogenesis and fasting glucose levels (Linn, Geyer et al. 1996; Linn, Santosa et al. 2000). Animal models also have shown that long-term high-protein diets impair insulin sensitivity and promote insulin resistance (Rossetti, Rothman et al. 1989). Previous study suggested that this insulin desensitization might be due to increased rate of β cell death (Schneider, Laube et al. 1996; Linn, Strate et al. 1999). However, these effects may depend on the source of protein.

Animal proteins versus plant proteins

The major difference between animal and plant proteins is the protein concentration per unit amount and the proportions of amino acids. Different amino acids could have distinct effects on glucose metabolism and insulin resistance. For example, arginine intake does not stimulate insulin secretion but attenuates the glucose rise when it was ingested with glucose (Gannon, Nuttall et al. 2002b). In contrast, oral glycine increases the serum insulin concentration and also attenuates the response to glucose (Gannon, Nuttall et al. 2002a). Different compositions of amino acids and their specific functions in animal and plant proteins may underlie their different effect on type 2 diabetes. As indicated earlier for strict vegetarians it is important to consume various types of food for mutual supplementation of essential amino acids, whereas complete proteins are found in animal food sources, including meat, poultry, fish, and dairy products.

Animal proteins. Research results from the Women's Health Study showed that red meat and animal protein intakes were significantly associated with an increased risk of type 2 diabetes, independent of total fat intake (Song, Manson et al. 2004). In the European Prospective Investigation into Cancer and Nutrition (EPIC)—NL study, animal proteins, which accounted for the majority of protein intake, were also associated with an increased risk of type 2 diabetes, independent of fat intake and meat or dairy intake (Sluijs, Beulens et al. 2010). These results indicated the deleterious effect of animal protein per se, rather than resulting from the effect of fat or other nutrients that are associated with animal protein.

Table 4.5 Studies of the Relation between Dietary Protein Intake and Insulin Resistance and Glucose Metabolism

Reference	Follow-up time	Study type	Population	Endpoint	Adjustment	Effect
McAuley et al. 2006 (McAuley, Smith et al. 2006)	12 months	RCT	93 over-weight insulin-resistant women	Various	Baseline variables	Substantial sustained improvement in insulin in the high-protein Zone diet group than the high-carbohydrate, high-fiber diet and the Atkins diet group
Samaha et al. 2003 (Samaha, Iqbal et al. 2003)	6 months	RCT	132 severely obese subjects	Obesity	Unadjusted	More improvement on insulin sensitivity in the low-carbohydrate diet (with significantly higher in take of protein) group than the low-fat diet group: $6 \pm 9\%$ versus $-3 \pm 8\%$
Stern et al. 2004 (Stern, Iqbal et al. 2004)	1 year	RCT	132 obese adults	Obesity	Age, race, sex, baseline body mass index, baseline caloric intake, and the presence or absence of hypertension, lipid-lowering therapy use, diabetes, active smoking, and sleep apnea	HbA1c improved more in the low-carbohydrate diet group (with significantly higher intake of protein) than the low-fat group: $-0.7 \pm 1.0\%$ versus $-0.1 \pm 1.6\%$
Sargrad et al. 2005 (Sargrad, Homko et al. 2005)	3 weeks	RCT	12 T2D patients	Various	Unadjusted	Standard protein group HbA1c and FPG decreased and insulin sensitivity increased.

(continued)

Table 4.5 Studies of the Relation between Dietary Protein Intake and Insulin Resistance and Glucose Metabolism (continued)

Reference	Follow-up time	Study type	Population	Endpoint	Adjustment	Effect
Gannon et al. 2003 (Gannon, Nuttall et al. 2003)	5 weeks	RCT	12 subjects with untreated T2D	Various	Unadjusted	High-protein diet (30%) versus control diet (15% protein, as recommended by several scientific organizations) Mean 24 h integrated glucose area responses: control 34.1 ± 7.2 mmol*h/L versus high-protein 21.0 ± 4.2 mmol*h/L Significant decrease of HbA1c in high-protein diet but not control diet Fasting insulin: control 104 ± 18 pmol/L versus high-protein 110 ± 21 pmol/L
Linn et al. 2000 (Linn, Santosa et al. 2000)	6 months	Cohort	18 subjects	Glucose metabolism	Unadjusted	High-protein versus normal-protein GSIS increased in high-protein group: 516 ± 45 pmol/L versus 305 ± 32 pmol/L Glucose threshold for insulin secretion: 4.2 ± 0.5 mmol/L versus 4.9 ± 0.3 mmol/L

Fish proteins are also of interest in terms of the effect on type 2 diabetes. Previously, the benefits from fish on reducing the incidence of type 2 diabetes were attributed to fish oil, especially polyunsaturated fatty acids. A meta-analysis, however, showed that daily intake of as much as 3 g fish oil has no protective effect on hyperglycemia in type 2 diabetes (Friedberg, Janssen et al. 1998). Since the ordinary consumption of fish provides much less fish oil than this level, the inverse association between fish intake and the risk of type 2 diabetes may be attributed to other components in fish. Fish proteins have been shown to affect glucose metabolism and insulin sensitivity. Animal studies showed that cod proteins, comparing with casein, improve fasting glucose tolerance and insulin sensitivity in peripheral tissues (Lavigne, Marette et al. 2000; Lavigne, Tremblay et al. 2001). Human studies also indicated that plasma insulin levels increased significantly less with a cod fillet meal compared with beef steak meal (Soucy and LeBlanc 1999). This suggests that insulin sensitivity was improved in the fish-feeding group, which may be a result of a greater rate of insulin-stimulated glucose uptake of myocytes when exposed to cod protein, compared with casein or soy proteins (Lavigne, Tremblay et al. 2001). It was also suggested that plasma amino acid profiles differ between a cod meal and red meat meal: arginine and lysine were higher with fish feeding and histidine was higher with beef feeding (Soucy and LeBlanc 1999). This may be another reason for the different effects between fish proteins and proteins from other animal sources on type 2 diabetes.

Plant proteins. In previous studies, plant proteins were not associated with incidence of type 2 diabetes (Sluijs, Beulens et al. 2010; Song, Manson et al. 2004). Some specific types of plant proteins, however, were shown to be associated with type 2 diabetes. Soy protein was indicated to be associated with a lower risk of type 2 diabetes in several studies (Davis, Iqbal et al. 2005; Villegas, Gao et al. 2008). Soy protein was suggested to ameliorate insulin resistance by improving peripheral insulin sensitivity and lowering postprandial plasma concentration in an animal study (Lavigne, Marette et al. 2000). Soy protein treatment was also suggested to increase PPARα and PPARγ expression in skeletal muscle compared with casein treatment (Wagner, Zhang et al. 2008). The protective effect of soy protein, however, is sometimes attributed to isoflavones or phytoestrogens in soy products (Jayagopal, Albertazzi et al. 2002; Mezei, Banz et al. 2003; Mueller et al. 2012). The detailed mechanism of the effect of soy protein still needs to be further studied.

Nut consumption has also been related to reduced risk of type 2 diabetes (Kendall, Josse et al. ; Jiang, Manson et al. 2002; Parker, Harnack et al. 2003; Jenkins, Hu et al. 2008). In the English language, a wide variety of edible dried fruits and seeds are called nuts, while only a small portion considered true nuts by biologists. Almonds, cashews, peanuts, and pistachios, do not meet the botanical definition of nuts. Nonetheless, all these have been clustered together due to their characteristics as good sources of unsaturated fatty acids, plant proteins, and other healthy nutritional profiles. Previous studies have shown that nut intake could lower postprandial glucose and insulin responses when consumed with other carbohydrate-rich foods (Jenkins, Kendall et al. 2006; Josse, Kendall et al. 2007). Whether the benefits from nuts are from plant proteins, unsaturated fatty acids, or other micronutrients still needs to be further investigated.

Protein supplementation

Gaining muscle or at least preservation of skeletal muscle mass is important for metabolic health, as skeletal muscle is the single largest site for blood glucose disposal and the second most important tissue contributing to thermogenesis, preceded by liver. The increase of muscle mass and glycolytic capacity of skeletal muscle could effectively offset insulin resistance and type 2 diabetes (LeBrasseur, Walsh et al.). Muscle anabolism occurs when proteins are consumed but is stimulated to a greater extent when resistance exercises are performed (Phillips 2004; Phillips, Hartman et al. 2005). The sources of common protein supplementation are whey protein and soy protein. Whey protein has been suggested to be more effective than muscle protein synthesis than soy protein (Phillips, Tang et al. 2009).

Molecular biology mechanisms

Besides the indirect effects of proteins on glucose metabolism and insulin resistance that were mentioned previously, direct effects of dietary proteins function through the interactions between its monomers—amino acids, and related receptors and downstream cascades of reactions. The role of amino acids on the metabolism and functioning of glucose and insulin has been recognized.

Perturbation of glucose intake

In the healthy human body, once the concentration of glucose in the circulation is elevated, blood insulin level increases to promote skeletal muscle and adipose tissue to take up glucose from the circulation, lowering the blood glucose level. In a human trial, elevated amino acids levels in plasma were shown to be able to induce skeletal muscle insulin resistance by inhibition of glucose transport and phosphorylation (Krebs, Krssak et al. 2002). This inhibitory effect of amino acids on insulin function was also indicated in cultured adipocytes and hepatocytes (Patti,

Brambilla et al. 1998; Takano, Usui et al. 2001). Amino acids were shown to be associated with phosphorylation of *insulin receptor substrate-1* (IRS-1) and impaired activation of *phosphoinositide 3-kinase* (PI3K) in vitro (Tremblay and Marette 2001), which activates GLUT-4 to uptake glucose from the circulation.

m-TOR pathway and insulin resistance

Previous studies have shown that amino acids participate in the phosphorylation of *70-kDa ribosomal S6 kinase* (RPS6KB1) and *eukaryotic initiation factor 4E-binding protein 1* (eIF4EBP1), which are located downstream of *mammalian target of rapamycin* (mTOR), modulating translation of proteins (Tremblay, Jacques et al. 2005; Tremblay, Lavigne et al. 2007). In the deprivation of amino acids in cell culture, the phosphorylation of RPS6KB1 and eIF4EBP1 declines dramatically, and reverses quickly after supplementation of amino acids (Iiboshi, Papst et al. 1999). The activation of mTOR and its downstream proteins RPS6KB1 and eIF4EBP1 by both insulin and amino acids inhibits PI3K by increased phosphorylation of IRS-1, thus leading to insulin resistance, since excessive serine-phosphorylated IRS-1 causes insulin resistance by blocking downstream signaling (PI3K) (Tremblay and Marette 2001). This pathway plays a significant role in the progress of insulin resistance under nutrient excess (Figure 4.4).

Hexosamine biosynthesis and insulin resistance

The hexosamine pathway in glucose metabolism has been related to insulin resistance and multiple adverse effects of hyperglycemia. Glutamine is the primary amino acid modulating glucose-induced decrease of maximal insulin responsiveness (Traxinger and Marshall 1989). It affects glucose transportation through activation of the *hexosamine pathway* (Marshall, Garvey et al. 1991). Activation of the hexosamine pathway could induce oxidative stress and deteriorate β cell function (Kaneto, Xu et al. 2001). Another mechanism of the effect of the hexosamine pathway on insulin resistance is that glucosamine, a product of the hexosamine pathway, causes a defect intrinsic to GLUT4 translocation and trafficking (Baron, Zhu et al. 1995).

Amino acids and hepatic glucose metabolism

Amino acids modulate endogenous glucose production in the liver. Some amino acids stimulate gluconeogenesis by acting as substrates, which are called *glucogenic amino acids* (Linn, Santosa et al. 2000). Gluconeogenesis is a metabolic pathway that generates glucose from noncarbohydrate carbon

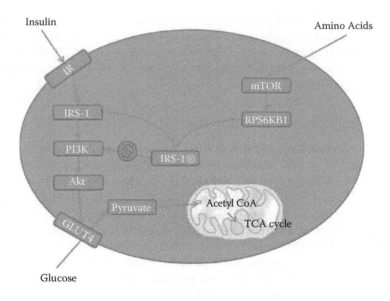

Figure 4.4 mTOR pathway and insulin resistance.

substrates. Amino acids can also stimulate glucagon and insulin secretion and affect endogenous glucose production, and modulate hepatic glucose metabolism by affecting the portal insulin/glucagon ratio (Floyd, Fajans et al. 1966; Roden, Perseghin et al. 1996; Linn, Santosa et al. 2000; Krebs, Brehm et al. 2003; Krebs 2005). While amino-acid-induced insulin secretion prevented a rise in plasma glucose concentration in healthy individuals, impaired insulin secretion unmasked this direct gluconeogenic effect of amino acids and resulted in overt hyperglycemia (Krebs, Brehm et al. 2003).

Conclusion

Dietary proteins can affect glucose metabolism and insulin resistance in the human body. This chapter introduced various effects of protein intake on glucose homeostasis and type 2 diabetes. Besides the intake of fat and carbohydrate, accounting for protein content in dietary recommendations for type 2 diabetes prevention and intervention may also be very important. The total effect of dietary proteins on glucose homeostasis and type 2 diabetes may involve a variety of metabolic pathways. Many of the conclusions regarding the relation between dietary protein and type 2 diabetes, however, are not conclusive and thus more studies are necessary.

References

Atkins, R. C. (2001). *Dr. Atkins' New Diet Revolution*. New York, Harper.

Baron, A. D., J. S. Zhu et al. (1995). "Glucosamine induces insulin resistance in vivo by affecting GLUT 4 translocation in skeletal muscle. Implications for glucose toxicity." *J Clin Invest* **96**(6): 2792–2801.

Batterham, R. L., H. Heffron et al. (2006). "Critical role for peptide YY in protein-mediated satiation and body-weight regulation." *Cell Metab* **4**(3): 223–233.

Blom, W. A., A. Lluch et al. (2006). "Effect of a high-protein breakfast on the post-prandial ghrelin response." *Am J Clin Nutr* **83**(2): 211–220.

Brinkworth, G. D., M. Noakes et al. (2004). "Long-term effects of a high-protein, low-carbohydrate diet on weight control and cardiovascular risk markers in obese hyperinsulinemic subjects." *Int J Obes Relat Metab Disord: J Int Assoc Study Obes* **28**(5): 661–670.

Bujnowski, D., P. Xun et al. (2011). "Longitudinal association between animal and vegetable protein intake and obesity among men in the United States: The Chicago Western Electric Study." *J Am Dietetic Assoc* **111**(8): 1150–1155 e1151.

Davis, J., M. J. Iqbal et al. (2005). "Soy protein influences the development of the metabolic syndrome in male obese ZDFxSHHF rats." *Horm Metab Res* **37**(5): 316–325.

de Koning, L., T. T. Fung et al. (2011). "Low-carbohydrate diet scores and risk of type 2 diabetes in men." *Am J Clin Nutr* **93**(4): 844–850.

Duc Son le, N. T., T. T. Hanh et al. (2005). "Anthropometric characteristics, dietary patterns and risk of type 2 diabetes mellitus in Vietnam." *J Am College Nutr* **24**(4): 229–234.

Evenepoel, P., D. Claus et al. (1999). "Amount and fate of egg protein escaping assimilation in the small intestine of humans." *Am J Physiol* **277**(5 Pt 1): G935–943.

Floyd, J. C., Jr., S. S. Fajans et al. (1966). "Stimulation of insulin secretion by amino acids." *J Clin Invest* **45**(9): 1487–1502.

Foster, G. D., H. R. Wyatt et al. (2003). "A randomized trial of a low-carbohydrate diet for obesity." *New Engl J Med* **348**(21): 2082–2090.

Friedberg, C. E., M. J. Janssen et al. (1998). "Fish oil and glycemic control in diabetes. A meta-analysis." *Diabetes Care* **21**(4): 494–500.

Gannon, M. C., F. Q. Nuttall et al. (2003). "An increase in dietary protein improves the blood glucose response in persons with type 2 diabetes." *Am J Clin Nutr* **78**(4): 734–741.

Gannon, M. C., J. A. Nuttall et al. (2002a). "The metabolic response to ingested glycine." *Am J Clin Nutr* **76**(6): 1302–1307.

Gannon, M. C., J. A. Nuttall et al. (2002b). "Oral arginine does not stimulate an increase in insulin concentration but delays glucose disposal." *Am J Clin Nutr* **76**(5): 1016–1022.

He, K., F. B. Hu et al. (2004). "Changes in intake of fruits and vegetables in relation to risk of obesity and weight gain among middle-aged women." *Int J Obes Relat Metab Disord: J Int Assoc Study Obes* **28**(12): 1569–1574.

Hu, F. B. (2005). "Protein, body weight, and cardiovascular health." *Am J Clin Nutr* **82**(1 Suppl): 242S–247S.

Iiboshi, Y., P. J. Papst et al. (1999). "Amino acid-dependent control of p70(s6k). Involvement of tRNA aminoacylation in the regulation." *J Biol Chem* **274**(2): 1092–1099.

Jayagopal, V., P. Albertazzi et al. (2002). "Beneficial effects of soy phytoestrogen intake in postmenopausal women with type 2 diabetes." *Diabetes Care* **25**(10): 1709–1714.

Jenkins, D. J., F. B. Hu et al. (2008). "Possible benefit of nuts in type 2 diabetes." *J Nutr* **138**(9): 1752S–1756S.

Jenkins, D. J., C. W. Kendall et al. (2006). "Almonds decrease postprandial glycemia, insulinemia, and oxidative damage in healthy individuals." *J Nutr* **136**(12): 2987–2992.

Jiang, R., J. E. Manson et al. (2002). "Nut and peanut butter consumption and risk of type 2 diabetes in women." *JAMA* **288**(20): 2554–2560.

Joo, N. S., Y. W. Park et al. (2011). "Application of protein-rich oriental diet in a community-based obesity control program." *Yonsei Med J* **52**(2): 249–256.

Josse, A. R., C. W. Kendall et al. (2007). "Almonds and postprandial glycemia—a dose-response study." *Metabolism* **56**(3): 400–404.

Kaneto, H., G. Xu et al. (2001). "Activation of the hexosamine pathway leads to deterioration of pancreatic beta-cell function through the induction of oxidative stress." *J Biol Chem* **276**(33): 31099–31104.

Kendall, C. W., A. R. Josse et al. "Nuts, metabolic syndrome and diabetes." *Br J Nutr* **104**(4): 465–473.

Krebs, M. (2005). "Amino acid-dependent modulation of glucose metabolism in humans." *Eur J Clin Invest* **35**(6): 351–354.

Krebs, M., A. Brehm et al. (2003). "Direct and indirect effects of amino acids on hepatic glucose metabolism in humans." *Diabetologia* **46**(7): 917–925.

Krebs, M., M. Krssak et al. (2002). "Mechanism of amino acid-induced skeletal muscle insulin resistance in humans." *Diabetes* **51**(3): 599–605.

Lavigne, C., A. Marette et al. (2000). "Cod and soy proteins compared with casein improve glucose tolerance and insulin sensitivity in rats." *Am J Physiol Endocrinol Metab* **278**(3): E491–500.

Lavigne, C., F. Tremblay et al. (2001). "Prevention of skeletal muscle insulin resistance by dietary cod protein in high fat-fed rats." *Am J Physiol Endocrinol Metab* **281**(1): E62–71.

LeBrasseur, N. K., K. Walsh et al. "Metabolic benefits of resistance training and fast glycolytic skeletal muscle." *Am J Physiol Endocrinol Metab* **300**(1): E3–10.

Linn, T., R. Geyer et al. (1996). "Effect of dietary protein intake on insulin secretion and glucose metabolism in insulin-dependent diabetes mellitus." *J Clin Endocrinol Metab* **81**(11): 3938–3943.

Linn, T., B. Santosa et al. (2000). "Effect of long-term dietary protein intake on glucose metabolism in humans." *Diabetologia* **43**(10): 1257–1265.

Linn, T., C. Strate et al. (1999). "Diet promotes beta-cell loss by apoptosis in prediabetic nonobese diabetic mice." *Endocrinology* **140**(8): 3767–3773.

Liu, S., J. E. Manson et al. (2000). "A prospective study of whole-grain intake and risk of type 2 diabetes mellitus in US women." *Am J Public Health* **90**(9): 1409–1415.

Liu, S., W. C. Willett et al. (2003). "Relation between changes in intakes of dietary fiber and grain products and changes in weight and development of obesity among middle-aged women." *Am J Clin Nutr* **78**(5): 920–927.

Luscombe, N. D., P. M. Clifton et al. (2002). "Effects of energy-restricted diets containing increased protein on weight loss, resting energy expenditure, and the thermic effect of feeding in type 2 diabetes." *Diabetes Care* **25**(4): 652–657.

Mahe, S., P. Marteau et al. (1994). "Intestinal nitrogen and electrolyte movements following fermented milk ingestion in man." *British J Nutr* **71**(2): 169–180.

Marshall, S., W. T. Garvey et al. (1991). "New insights into the metabolic regulation of insulin action and insulin resistance: Role of glucose and amino acids." *FASEB J* **5**(15): 3031–3036.

McAuley, K. A., C. M. Hopkins et al. (2005). "Comparison of high-fat and high-protein diets with a high-carbohydrate diet in insulin-resistant obese women." *Diabetologia* **48**(1): 8–16.

McAuley, K. A., K. J. Smith et al. (2006). "Long-term effects of popular dietary approaches on weight loss and features of insulin resistance." *Int J Obesity* **30**(2): 342–349.

Mezei, O., W. J. Banz et al. (2003). "Soy isoflavones exert antidiabetic and hypolipidemic effects through the PPAR pathways in obese Zucker rats and murine RAW 264.7 cells." *J Nutr* **133**(5): 1238–1243.

Montignac, M. (2003). *Je mange donc je maigris ... et je reste mince.* Paris, J'ai lu.

Mueller, N. T., A. O. Odegaard et al. "Soy intake and risk of type 2 diabetes in Chinese Singaporeans," *Euro. J. Nutr.* **51**(8): 1033–1040.

Nair, K. S., D. Halliday et al. (1983). "Thermic response to isoenergetic protein, carbohydrate or fat meals in lean and obese subjects." *Clin Sci (Lond)* **65**(3): 307–312.

Parker, E. D., L. J. Harnack et al. (2003). "Nut consumption and risk of type 2 diabetes." *JAMA* **290**(1): 38–39; author reply 39–40.

Patti, M. E., E. Brambilla et al. (1998). "Bidirectional modulation of insulin action by amino acids." *J Clin Invest* **101**(7): 1519–1529.

Petzke, K. J., C. Riese et al. (2007). "Short-term, increasing dietary protein and fat moderately affect energy expenditure, substrate oxidation and uncoupling protein gene expression in rats." *J Nutr Biochem* **18**(6): 400–407.

Phillips, S. M. (2004). "Protein requirements and supplementation in strength sports." *Nutrition* **20**(7–8): 689–695.

Phillips, S. M., J. W. Hartman et al. (2005). "Dietary protein to support anabolism with resistance exercise in young men." *J Am College Nutr* **24**(2): 134S–139S.

Phillips, S. M., J. E. Tang et al. (2009). "The role of milk- and soy-based protein in support of muscle protein synthesis and muscle protein accretion in young and elderly persons." *J Am College Nutr* **28**(4): 343–354.

Promintzer, M. and M. Krebs (2006). "Effects of dietary protein on glucose homeostasis." *Curr Opin Clin Nutr Metab Care* **9**(4): 463–468.

Remer, T., K. Pietrzik et al. (1996). "A moderate increase in daily protein intake causing an enhanced endogenous insulin secretion does not alter circulating levels or urinary excretion of dehydroepiandrosterone sulfate." *Metabolism* **45**(12): 1483–1486.

Roden, M., G. Perseghin et al. (1996). "The roles of insulin and glucagon in the regulation of hepatic glycogen synthesis and turnover in humans." *J Clin Invest* **97**(3): 642–648.

Rossetti, L., D. L. Rothman et al. (1989). "Effect of dietary protein on in vivo insulin action and liver glycogen repletion." *Am J Physiol* **257**(2 Pt 1): E212–219.

Samaha, F. F., N. Iqbal et al. (2003). "A low-carbohydrate as compared with a low-fat diet in severe obesity." *New Engl J Med* **348**(21): 2074–2081.

Sargrad, K. R., C. Homko et al. (2005). "Effect of high protein vs high carbohydrate intake on insulin sensitivity, body weight, hemoglobin A1c, and blood pressure in patients with type 2 diabetes mellitus." *J Am Dietetic Assoc* **105**(4): 573–580.

Schneider, K., H. Laube et al. (1996). "A diet enriched in protein accelerates diabetes manifestation in NOD mice." *Acta Diabetol* **33**(3): 236–240.

Sluijs, I., J. W. Beulens et al. (2010). "Dietary intake of total, animal, and vegetable protein and risk of type 2 diabetes in the European Prospective Investigation into Cancer and Nutrition (EPIC)-NL study." *Diabetes Care* **33**(1): 43–48.

Soenen, S. and M. S. Westerterp-Plantenga (2010). "Changes in body fat percentage during body weight stable conditions of increased daily protein intake vs. control." *Physiol Behav* **101**(5): 635–638.

Song, Y., J. E. Manson et al. (2004). "A prospective study of red meat consumption and type 2 diabetes in middle-aged and elderly women: The women's health study." *Diabetes Care* **27**(9): 2108–2115.

Soucy, J. and J. LeBlanc (1999). "The effects of a beef and fish meal on plasma amino acids, insulin and glucagon levels." *Nutr Res* **19**(1): 17–24.

Spiller, G. A., C. D. Jensen et al. (1987). "Effect of protein dose on serum glucose and insulin response to sugars." *Am J Clin Nutr* **46**(3): 474–480.

Stern, L., N. Iqbal et al. (2004). "The effects of low-carbohydrate versus conventional weight loss diets in severely obese adults: One-year follow-up of a randomized trial." *Ann Intern Med* **140**(10): 778–785.

Takano, A., I. Usui et al. (2001). "Mammalian target of rapamycin pathway regulates insulin signaling via subcellular redistribution of insulin receptor substrate 1 and integrates nutritional signals and metabolic signals of insulin." *Mol Cell Biol* **21**(15): 5050–5062.

Tannous dit El Khoury, D., O. Obeid et al. (2006). "Variations in postprandial ghrelin status following ingestion of high-carbohydrate, high-fat, and high-protein meals in males." *Ann Nutr Metab* **50**(3): 260–269.

Traxinger, R. R. and S. Marshall (1989). "Role of amino acids in modulating glucose-induced desensitization of the glucose transport system." *J Biol Chem* **264**(35): 20910–20916.

Tremblay, F., H. Jacques et al. (2005). "Modulation of insulin action by dietary proteins and amino acids: Role of the mammalian target of rapamycin nutrient sensing pathway." *Curr Opin Clin Nutr Metab Care* **8**(4): 457–462.

Tremblay, F., C. Lavigne et al. (2007). "Role of dietary proteins and amino acids in the pathogenesis of insulin resistance." *Annu Rev Nutr* **27**: 293–310.

Tremblay, F. and A. Marette (2001). "Amino acid and insulin signaling via the mTOR/p70 S6 kinase pathway: A negative feedback mechanism leading to insulin resistance in skeletal muscle cells." *J Biol Chem* **276**(41): 38052–38060.

Villegas, R., Y. T. Gao et al. (2008). "Legume and soy food intake and the incidence of type 2 diabetes in the Shanghai Women's Health Study." *Am J Clin Nutr* **87**(1): 162–167.

Wagner, J. D., L. Zhang et al. (2008). "Effects of soy protein and isoflavones on insulin resistance and adiponectin in male monkeys." *Metabolism***57**(7 Suppl 1): S24–31.

Wang, E. T., L. de Koning et al. (2010). "Higher protein intake is associated with diabetes risk in South Asian Indians: The Metabolic Syndrome and Atherosclerosis in South Asians Living in America (MASALA) study." *J Am College Nutr* **29**(2): 130–135.

Weigle, D. S., P. A. Breen et al. (2005). "A high-protein diet induces sustained reductions in appetite, ad libitum caloric intake, and body weight despite compensatory changes in diurnal plasma leptin and ghrelin concentrations." *Am J Clin Nutr* **82**(1): 41–48.

Wolever, T. M., S. Hamad et al. (1997). "Low dietary fiber and high protein intakes associated with newly diagnosed diabetes in a remote aboriginal community." *Am J Clin Nutr* **66**(6): 1470–1474.

chapter five

Micronutrients and type 2 diabetes

Simin Liu, MD, ScD
University of California, Los Angeles (UCLA)

Yiqing Song, MD, ScD
Brigham and Women's Hospital, Harvard Medical School

Contents

Introduction

Given the increasing incidence of type 2 diabetes, the identification of effective and safe preventive measures that offer even modest reductions in incidence could have a significant public health impact. One promising but as-yet-unproven nutritional strategy for the prevention of diabetes or diabetic complications is increased micronutrients intake (American Diabetes Association 1998). Indeed, considerable uncertainty exists regarding the efficacy of these agents. While a large body of basic biologic data suggest that they reduce oxidative damage to the endothelial membrane and thus improve endothelial function and insulin sensitivity (American Diabetes Association 1997; Colewell 1997), available epidemiologic and clinical data provide equivocal information regarding their efficacy in reducing the risk of type 2 diabetes. When evaluating the efficacy of agents with small-to-moderate effects using data from observational studies, biases due to misclassification and/or residual confounding by other healthy behaviors associated with the use of these agents cannot be excluded. Randomized, double-blind, placebo-controlled trials are the best option for establishing (or refuting) potential causal associations. One major gap in the current knowledge base is the lack of long-term, randomized, and primary prevention trials directly evaluating the clinical efficacy of specific micronutrients for the primary prevention of type 2 diabetes.

Despite the lack of "gold-standard" evidence linking use of micronutrients to the prevention of chronic disease, considerable attention in the lay press and the scientific literature combined with ready access have led to their widespread usage. One national survey indicated that 32% of men and 45% of women regularly use nutritional supplements (Kim, Williamson et al. 1993), and the doses of supplementation often exceed the recommended dietary allowance (RDA) (McDonald 1986). US consumers now spend more than $12 billion per year on dietary supplements (Zeisel 1999). With national sales increased from $260 million in 1988 to $338 million in 1993, vitamin C and vitamin E are the two most popular single-product supplements sold in the United States (Lerner 1998). In this chapter, we will review the available literature concerning the efficacy of vitamin E, vitamin C, β-carotene, vitamin D, magnesium, folic acid and other B vitamins, and multivitamins in reducing the risk of type 2 diabetes.

Antioxidants

Basic biologic data

Considerable evidence supports the theory that free radicals play an important role in the development of many chronic degenerative diseases of aging, including type 2 diabetes (Ames, Shigenaga et al. 1993; Halliwell 1994). Highly reactive free radicals can oxidize and damage such essential molecules as DNA, proteins, and lipids (Halliwell 1994), and accumulation of damaged, oxidized, and dysfunctional peptides is one of the most fundamental manifestations of aging (Ames, Shigenaga et al. 1993). To guard against oxidative damage caused by free radicals, two major defense mechanisms—the enzymatic (intracellular defense) and the non-enzymatic (intercellular defense)—are found in the human body. The intracellular defense comprises catalases such as proteasome, glutathione peroxidase, and superoxide dismutase (Rivett 1985a; Rivett 1985b), whereas antioxidants such as vitamin E and vitamin C constitute the primary intercellular defense against free radicals (Frei 1994a; Frei 1994b). In laboratory research, vitamin C, vitamin E, and other antioxidants have been shown to prevent tissue damage by trapping organic free radicals and/or deactivating excited oxygen molecules, which are by-products of many metabolic functions (Packer 1991). This antioxidant activity may slow or prevent atherosclerotic plaque formation by inhibiting oxidation of low-density lipoprotein cholesterol (LDL), thus protecting the vascular wall from oxidized LDL and other cytotoxic oxidative products (Steinberg 1991). Vitamin E may also modify platelet activity,[21-23] reduce thrombotic potential,[24] and modify vascular reactivity[25-27] via antioxidant-related modifications in prostaglandin metabolism and nitric oxide production.

Insulin resistance and progressive pancreatic ß-cell dysfunction are well-established defects in the pathogenesis of type 2 DM (Kahn 1994). Tissue resistance to the action of insulin is believed to be a common antecedent to both type 2 DM and atherosclerotic disease (Pyorala 1979; Stout 1990; Stern 1995). Much research has also demonstrated that both insulin resistance and hyperglycemia increase oxidative stress and thus accelerate the atherosclerotic process. The manifestations of dyslipidemia and hemodynamic risk factors for CVD are collectively termed the insulin resistant syndrome.[32]

Several mechanisms, including nonenzymatic glycation of protein, glucose auto-oxidation, and increased polyol pathway activity, may account for increased oxidative stress in diabetic individuals (Figure 5.1) (Giugliano, Ceriello et al. 1996; Paolisso and Giugliano 1996; Bloomgarden 1997). Increased nonenzymatic glycation of LDLs has been shown to decrease receptor-mediated uptake and catabolism of LDLs (Lyons 1992), which leads to the transformation of macrophages into foam cells, an effect also

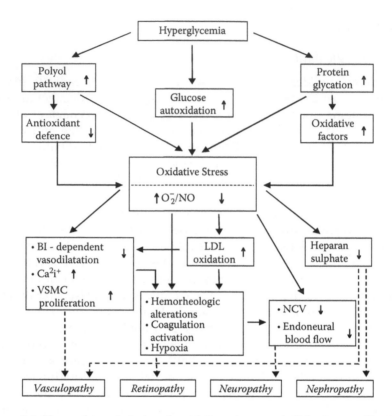

Figure 5.1 Hyperglycemia-induced oxidative stress and diabetic complications. (Modified from Giugliano, Ceriello et al. *Diabetes Care* **19**(3): 257–267.)

shared by oxidized LDLs. With regard to diabetic complications, advanced glycosylation end products (AGEs) have been shown to influence vascular structure. Hyperglycemia can affect all stages of coagulation, including fibrinolysis and platelet and endothelial function (Ceriello, Giugliano et al. 1991). Glucose autoxidation produces superoxide anion (O_2^-), hydroxyl radical (OH-), and hydrogen peroxide (H_2O_2). All these free radicals can damage the endothelial membrane through cross-linking and fragmentation. The formation of AGEs supplies more free radicals, further aggravating oxidative stress. This process has been termed autoxidative glycosylation (Baynes and Thorpe 1999). Even mildly elevated glucose levels can cause an increase in intracellular sorbitol and fructose levels through increased activity of aldose reductase and sorbitol dehydrogenase (Giugliano, Ceriello et al. 1996) via the so-called polyol pathway. Increased substrate flux through the polyol pathway decreases the ratio of NADPH to NADP+ and increases the cytosolic NADH-to-NAD+ ratio, inhibiting the body's natural antioxidant defense (Williamson, Chang et al. 1993).

Pancreatic ß-cells have been characterized by low concentrations of radical scavengers (Jain and Palmer 1997), and are thus susceptible to damage from free radicals (Beales, Williams et al. 1994). In experimental studies, diabetes can be induced by free radicals, and antioxidants can prevent this induction by acting as free-radical scavengers (Oberley 1988). In animal models such as Sprague-Dawley rats, the higher the serum insulin level, the greater the decrease of catalase activity (Xu and Badr 1999). Several research groups have shown that an increase in serum insulin concentrations maintained for 1 week significantly inhibited catalase activity, leading to a net accumulation of hydrogen peroxide (H_2O_2) and increased production of superoxide anion and hydroxyl radical (Kashiwagi, Shinozaki et al. 1999a, 1999b; Xu and Badr 1999). In particular, increased oxidative stress (i.e., an increase in the ratio of oxidized glutathione [GSSG] to plasma reduced glutathione [GSH]) may directly affect glucose tolerance through adverse changes in glucose transport that result from lipid peroxidation of the cell membranes (Oberley 1988; Caballero 1993). Studies in both rats (Ammon, Klumpp et al. 1989) and humans (Paolisso, Giugliano et al. 1992; Paolisso, D'Amore et al. 1993) have found that changes in the ratio of plasma-oxidized glutathione to plasma-reduced glutathione can also affect β-cell insulin secretion. Recent studies also suggest that even among apparently healthy, nondiabetic, insulin-resistant individuals, hyperinsulinemia reduces degradation of oxidized protein molecules and facilitates protein oxidation by increasing steady-state levels of oxidative stress, independent of the state of hyperglycemia (Facchini, Hua et al. 2000). Paolisso et al. have suggested that antioxidants such as vitamin E may protect the integrity of plasma membranes by increasing GSH concentration and thus improving insulin action and glucose transport activities (Paolisso, D'Amore et al. 1993).

Dietary antioxidants and type 2 diabetes

No randomized trial has yet been conducted to examine the efficacy of antioxidant vitamins for the primary prevention of type 2 DM in free-living human populations. As discussed above, however, considerable experimental and observational data suggest that increased oxidative stress plays an important role in the pathogenesis of diabetes and its complications (Chisolm, Irwin et al. 1992; Paolisso, D'Amore et al. 1993; Dandona, Thusu et al. 1996; Giugliano, Ceriello et al. 1996; Paolisso and Giugliano 1996; Bloomgarden 1997; Facchini, Hua et al. 2000; Facchini, Humphreys et al. 2000). Many small-scale clinical studies have reported that increased free radical activity and high lipid oxidation are associated with impaired glucose disposal in the peripheral tissues and exacerbated diabetic complications (Paolisso, D'Amore et al. 1993; Golay and Felber 1994). Even among apparently healthy, nondiabetic individuals, the greater the insulin resistance among individuals, the higher their total plasma concentration of lipid hydroperoxides and oxidized LDL, suggesting a potential protective role of antioxidants in reducing the risk of type 2 DM (Carantoni, Abbasi et al. 1998; Facchini, Hua et al. 2000; Facchini, Humphreys et al. 2000). In a recent study of 36 apparently healthy volunteers, Facchini et al. reported a statistically significant inverse relation between insulin resistance and plasma levels of lipid-soluble vitamins, including α-tocopherol ($r = -0.36$, $p = 0.04$) (Facchini, Humphreys et al. 2000). Further, in a recent trial of 10 healthy individuals and 15 with type 2 DM, administration of vitamin E (900 mg per day for 4 months) was found to improve insulin sensitivity and reduce oxidative stress (Paolisso, D'Amore et al. 1993). Taken together, these basic biologic and clinical data suggest that inadequate antioxidant vitamins contribute to a decrease in plasma concentration of antioxidants, which in turn impairs the ability of insulin to stimulate glucose disposal by peripheral tissues. Insulin resistance results in an increase in lipid peroxidation and free-radical productions, further depleting plasma antioxidants and aggravating insulin resistance and hyperglycemia. This self-perpetuating cycle may eventually cause the failure of pancreatic β-cells to produce insulin in response to glucose, leading to clinical diabetes.

Much of the epidemiologic evidence supporting the role of antioxidants in prevention of type 2 DM has been indirect. Overall, higher intake of antioxidant-rich fruits, vegetables, and whole grains has been related to lower risk of type 2 DM. Ecological studies have suggested that populations with a high intake of animal products but a low intake of dietary antioxidants from fruits, vegetables, and whole grains tend to have high prevalence of type 2 DM (Harris 1985; Manson and Spelsberg 1994). However, such comparisons among populations cannot provide definitive answers, because this approach cannot fully adjust for other important factors such as exercise and other lifestyle behaviors that may confound the diet–diabetes association. Moreover, since the diagnosis of DM is often followed by alterations in diet, physical activity, and other lifestyle practices, the value of retrospective studies is limited. Prospective cohort studies are better suited to evaluate the role of diet in the development of type 2 DM because diets are assessed prior to the outcome and reporting of intake is not biased by a recent diagnosis of diabetes. In several prospective assessments of diet and type 2 DM conducted in the United States and Europe, increased consumption of vegetables has been associated with reduced risk of type 2 DM (Snowdon and Phillips 1985; Colditz, Manson et al. 1992; Feskens, Virtanen et al. 1995). In a study of 25,698 white Seventh Day Adventist adults followed for 21 years, vegetarians had a substantially lower risk of diabetes than nonvegetarians (Snowdon and Phillips 1985). In a study of 84,360 female nurses followed for 6 years, Colditz et al. observed an inverse association between intake of vegetables and risk of type 2 DM among women with BMIs <29 (Colditz, Manson et al. 1992). Specifically, women in the highest quintile of vegetable intake (>2.9 servings/day) had a relative risk of 0.76 (95% CI, 0.50–1.16) compared with those consuming <1.2 servings/day. In a cohort of 814 European men followed for 10 years, higher consumption of vegetables and legumes was inversely associated with glucose intolerance, as indicated by the 2-hour glucose level. In a randomized trial of 577 individuals with impaired glucose tolerance conducted in Da Qing, China, those assigned to a diet with more vegetables had a 24% lower incidence of type 2 DM than the control group during 6 years of follow-up (Pan, Cao et al. 1997). More recently, two prospective cohort studies of women reported an inverse association between intake of whole-grain foods and risk of type 2 DM. In the Iowa Women's Health Study, Meyer and colleagues reported a significant inverse association between intake of whole grains and risk of type 2 DM among 35,988 women aged 55 to 69 years followed for 6 years (Meyer, K., Kushi, L.H., Jacobs, D.R., Slavin, J., Sellers, T.A., Folsom A.R., 2000). After adjusting for known risk factors, the relative risk of type 2 DM was 0.79 (95% CI, 0.64–0.96) comparing the two extreme quintiles of whole grain intake. In the Nurses' Health Study, we reported strong dose-response relationships of intake of whole grains and their major food sources to risk of type 2 DM among 75,521 women aged 38 to 63 years followed for 10 years (Liu, Manson et al. 2000). Comparing the highest and lowest quintiles of intake, the age- and energy-adjusted relative risks were 0.62 (95% CI, 0.53–0.71; P for trend < 0.0001). After additional adjustment for BMI and other potential risk factors, these associations were attenuated but remained significant: comparing the two extreme quintiles of whole grain intake, the relative risk of type 2 DM was 0.73 (95% CI, 0.63–0.89; P for trend < 0.0001).

Only a few prospective studies have examined directly the relations between dietary intakes of antioxidant vitamins and diabetes incidence. In a 20-year prospective study of Dutch and Finnish adults, Feskens and colleagues found similar inverse relations between dietary vitamin C and glucose intolerance or incidence of diabetes (Feskens, Virtanen et al. 1995). In the National Health and Nutrition Examination Survey I Epidemiologic Follow-up Study of 9573 men and women, Ford reported that in comparison to nonsupplement users, those who used vitamin supplements had a 24% (95% CI, 7%–37%) lower risk of developing diabetes over 20 years of follow-up (Ford 2001). In particular, participants who used vitamins regularly and consistently over a 10-year period had a larger reduction in risk (RR, 0.47; 95% CI, 0.27–0.81) than those who used vitamins irregularly, suggesting a dose-response relation.

Serum levels of antioxidants, intermediate markers, and risk of type 2 diabetes

The bioavailability of antioxidants can be reflected by their plasma concentrations (Michaud, Giovannucci et al. 1998; van het Hof, Brouwer et al. 1999). It is thus important to evaluate directly the relation between plasma levels of antioxidants and risk of type 2 DM. However, plasma concentration of antioxidants can be affected not only by intake of dietary antioxidants but also by genetic and lifestyle factors and by other dietary factors. Therefore, a useful biomarker should reflect long-term intake over time (time integration) because the etiology of type 2 DM may well be related to long-term deficiency of dietary antioxidants. In this regard, plasma levels of vitamin E correlate very well with dietary intakes and supplements, after appropriate adjustment for confounding factors such as age, sex, smoking status, and blood lipids (Willett 1998). In particular, in metabolic studies conducted among individuals with type 2 DM, vitamin E supplementation significantly reduced plasma levels of glycosylated hemoglobin (Ceriello, Giugliano et al. 1991), reflecting improved metabolic control. Recently, Salonen et al. reported a strong independent association between low levels of plasma vitamin E and excess risk of type 2 DM among 944 men followed for 4 years in Eastern Finland (Salonen, Nyyssonen et al. 1995). In cross-sectional studies, plasma levels of antioxidants have also been related to prevalence of diabetes or glucose intolerance (Will and Byers 1996; Rock, Jahnke et al. 1997; Ford, Will et al. 1999), lending further support to the proposition that maintaining certain physiological levels of antioxidants plays an important role in the prevention of type 2 DM. In a small nested-case-control study of 106 Finns with diabetes and 201 controls, serum alpha-tocopherol was not significantly related to diabetes incidence after adjustment for known diabetes risk factors (Reunanen, Knekt et al. 1998). In a review of 30 published studies, Will and Byers found that diabetic individuals tend to have at least 30% lower plasma vitamin C level than people without diabetes (Will and Byers 1996), suggesting a potential direct link between plasma vitamin C and glucose level. More recently, in a large population-based study in Europe, Sargeant and colleagues reported a significant inverse association between plasma vitamin C levels and HbA1c (Sargeant, Wareham et al. 2000). Observational data, however, cannot definitively determine whether low plasma concentrations of antioxidants precede the onset of diabetes, and thus cause it whether the low concentrations were consequences of latent diabetes at the time of the measurement, or whether the associations are confounded by other dietary or lifestyle factors.

In summary, considerable evidence from basic biologic, clinical, and epidemiologic research suggest that antioxidants—particularly, vitamin E or vitamin C—may be important agents in reducing the risk of type 2

DM. However, there have been few clinical trials on vitamin supplements for primary prevention of type 2 DM. Secondary analyses of randomized clinical trials on cardiovascular events and cancers found no significant effects of vitamin E or β-carotene supplementation on the incidence of type 2 DM (Liu, Lee et al. 2006; Song, Cook et al. 2009). Vitamin C is a potent water-soluble antioxidant and can effectively scavenge several reactive species and regenerate tocopherols and tocotrenols from their respective radical species (Padayatty, Katz et al. 2003). Vitamin C may also have a role in the energy-dependent release of insulin from pancreatic islets (Wells, Dou et al. 1995). Some small- and short-term randomized trials have been conducted among patients with type 2 diabetes; some reported that vitamin C supplementation (1–2 g/day) reduced oxidative stress and improved endothelial function in diabetic patients (Padayatty, Katz et al. 2003). Further, a recent trial has shown suggestive evidence for vitamin C (500 mg/day) in preventing type 2 diabetes among women at high risk of cardiovascular disease (Song, Cook et al. 2009). Due to limited data from randomized trials, these data alone are inadequate to answer whether antioxidants have a long-term effect on risk of type 2 DM.

Homocysteine and folic acid/vitamin B_6/vitamin B_{12}

Homocysteine is a sulfur-containing amino acid formed during the metabolism of methionine, an essential amino acid derived from dietary protein. When excess methionine is present, homocysteine is linked with serine to form cystathionine in a reaction catalyzed by cystathionine ß-synthase, a vitamin B_6-dependent enzyme (Figure 5.2). Otherwise, homocysteine is recycled to methionine by acquiring a methyl group from N^5-methyltetrahydrofolate in a reaction catalyzed by the vitamin B_{12}-dependent enzyme methionine synthase (Welch and Loscalzo 1998). Homocysteine impairs the function of endothelial cell membranes (Starkebaum and Harlan 1986; Nappo, De Rosa et al. 1999), oxidizes low-density lipoprotein (Heinecke, Kawamura et al. 1993), promotes proliferation of smooth muscle cells (Lentz and Sadler 1991), and adversely affects hemostatic and coagulation factors. Homocysteine has also been shown to reduce endothelial cell-associated tPA activity in vitro (Hajjar 1993). Elevated levels of homocysteine induce increased generation of hydrogen peroxide and cellular growth factors such as platelet-derived growth factor in cultures of endothelial cells and smooth muscle cells (Clopath, Smith et al. 1976; Parasarathy 1987). It also induces oxidation of LDL and enhances the binding of lipoprotein(a) to fibrin (Harpel, Chang et al. 1992). Homocysteine may also be involved in inflammatory processes leading to atherosclerosis (Bazzano, L.A., Reynolds, K., Holder, K.N., He, J., 2006). One possible unifying hypothesis is that elevated levels of homocysteine result in the formation of oxygen-free radicals that, in turn, cause vascular

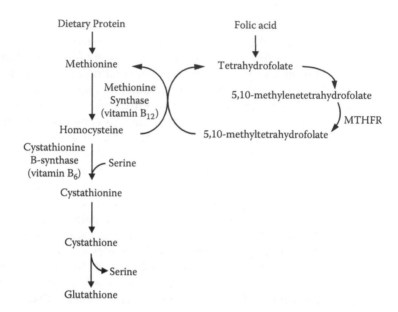

Figure 5.2 Interactions of folic acid, vitamin B_6, and vitamin B_{12} with homocysteine metabolism.

damage and endothelial dysfunction, proliferation of smooth muscle cells, impaired vascular reactivity, and increased thrombogenicity (Smolin, L., Benevenga, N., 1982).

Homocysteinemia may promote insulin resistance and β-cell dysfunction through its adverse metabolic effects, ultimately contributing to the pathogenesis of type 2 DM and associated complications (Welch and Loscalzo 1998; Hofmann, Lalla et al. 2001; Weiss, Heydrick et al. 2003). Several lines of evidence from both in vitro and in vivo studies support this hypothesis. First, homocysteinemia directly elicits oxidative stress by increasing reactive oxygen species production and diminishing intracellular antioxidant defense (Weiss, Heydrick et al. 2003). Experimental studies suggested that oxidative stress interferes with insulin signaling and impairs pancreatic β-cell insulin secretion (Evans, Goldfine et al. 2003; Ceriello and Motz, 2004), thereby accelerating the progression from insulin resistance to overt type 2 DM. Second, elevated levels of homocysteine promote systemic inflammation via the activation of a cascade of inflammatory pathways including IL-6, TNF-α, and adhesion molecules (Hofmann, Lalla et al. 2001). Low-grade chronic inflammation, as reflected by elevated circulating levels of inflammatory cytokines, may promote insulin resistance in liver, skeletal muscle, and vascular endothelium (Hotamisligil, Shargill et al. 1993; Uysal, Wiesbrock et al. 1997). Last, homocysteine can exert its damaging effects on the endothelium through mechanisms involving impaired nitric-oxide-dependent vasodilation, endothelial toxicity and injury, oxidative stress, and systemic inflammation (Stamler, Osborne et al. 1993; Weiss, Heydrick et al. 2003). The resultant endothelial dysfunction, especially in the capillary and arteriolar endothelium, can reduce insulin delivery to insulin-sensitive peripheral tissues, which in turn impairs insulin-mediated glucose metabolism (Pinkney, Stehouwer et al. 1997; Caballero 2003; Kim, Montagnani et al. 2006). Collectively, it seems plausible to speculate that elevated homocysteine levels may play an etiologic role in the development of insulin resistance and type 2 DM primarily by promoting oxidative stress, systemic inflammation, and endothelial dysfunction. (Abbasi, Facchini et al. 1999; Sheu, Lee et al. 2000; Godsland, Rosankiewicz et al. 2001; Meigs, Jacques et al. 2001; van Etten, de Koning et al. 2002; van Guldener and Stehouwer 2002; Fonseca, Fink et al. 2003; Hunter-Lavin, Hudson et al. 2004; Cho, Lim et al. 2005; Mangoni, Sherwood et al. 2005; Title, Ur et al. 2006; Hajer, van der Graaf et al. 2007; Song, Cook et al. 2009; van Etten, de Koning et al. 2002; Hunter-Lavin, Hudson et al. 2004; Spoelstra-de, Brouwer et al. 2004; Bazzano, Reynolds et al. 2006).

Treatment of hyperhomocysteinemia

Folate, pyridoxine (vitamin B_6), and cyanocobalamin (vitamin B_{12}) are cofactors in the enzymatic pathways of homocysteine metabolism (Figure 5.2). Deficiencies of each of these vitamins can result in elevated homocysteine levels (Smolin and Benevenga 1982; Kang, Wong et al. 1987; Brattstrom, Israelsson et al. 1990; Brattstrom 1996). Folic acid appears to have the strongest inverse association with homocysteine levels and reduces homocysteine even when given alone (Ubbink, Vermaak et al. 1994). Recently, a direct inverse association between serum folate and fatal CHD risk was observed in 5,056 men and women. Those in the lowest quartile of serum folate, corresponding to a folic acid intake of 200 µg or lower, had a 69% increased risk of fatal CHD compared to those in the highest quartile, corresponding to a folic acid intake of 400 µg or higher (Brattstrom 1996). Inadequate plasma concentrations of one or more B vitamins appeared to contribute to 67% of the cases of hyperhomocysteinemia in an elderly population in the Framingham Study (Selhub, Jacques et al. 1993).

Intervention studies have demonstrated decreases in plasma homocysteine after administration of 650 to 10,000 µg of folic acid (Brattstrom 1996). All subjects in these studies had normal concentrations of folate, vitamin B_{12}, and vitamin B_6 before the intervention. Large doses of folic acid do not appear to be necessary to lower plasma homocysteine levels. The reduction obtained from 5000 µg/d of folic acid is equivalent to that from 1000 µg/d, and a dose of 650 µg/d was sufficient to lower homocysteine levels by 42% in normal subjects with initially elevated levels of homocysteine. In a study by O'Keefe et al., significant reductions in homocysteine levels were obtained by increasing consumption of folic acid from 200 µg/day to 400 µg/day (O'Keefe, Bailey et al. 1995). At present, 88% of the US population is estimated to consume less than 400 µg/day of folic acid and, even with the folic acid fortification of foods, approximately 76% of this population will consume less than 400 µg/day. Thus, the role for intervention continues to be high. Selhub's group has estimated that even with folic acid fortification, at least 20.1% of Americans over 65 years of age will have homocysteine levels greater than 14.0 µmol/L (Tucker, Mahnken et al. 1996).

Vitamin B_6 plays a crucial role in reducing abnormal homocysteine responses after a methionine load (Brattstrom 1996). Abnormal responses to a methionine load are much more common among individuals with cardiovascular (CVD) than among controls. Vitamin B_{12} lowers homocysteine levels primarily in the setting of B_{12} deficiency, but has also been shown to lower fasting homocysteine levels in those without B_{12} deficiency. Given these data and the not uncommon occurrence of nutritional deficiencies of the B-complex vitamins in the elderly—5% of the Framingham population had insufficient levels of vitamin B_{12} not related to pernicious anemia (Lindebaum, Rosenburg et al. 1994)—it therefore would be important to test a combined supplement of all three vitamins in the prevention of type 2 DM.

Homocysteine and cardiovascular disease (CVD)

Based on the earlier observations of vascular disease in patients with homocystinuria, McCully (1969) first proposed a hypothesis that increased homocysteiene concentrations might be causally related to CVD risk in the general population (McCully 1969). Homocystinuria is a rare autosomal recessive disorder, which is usually caused by homozygous deficiency of cystathionine β-synthase, an enzyme required in methionine metabolism for the conversion of homocysteine to cystathionine. Patients with untreated homocystinuria have at least a ten-fold higher level of homocysteine concentrations than healthy subjects, and they are prone to develop premature atherosclerosis and thromboembolism in early life. Accumulating data from epidemiological studies suggested that elevated homocysteine levels are very common in the general population and individuals with even moderate elevated levels of homocysteine (>16 umol/L) have small-to-moderate increased risks of CVD (Stampfer, Malinow et al. 1992). Intervention studies have shown that modest amounts of folic acid, vitamin B_6, and/or vitamin B_{12}, as well as vitamin E or vitamin C, reduce homocysteine levels (Brattstrom, Israelsson et al. 1988; Brattstrom

1996; Nappo, De Rosa et al. 1999). The mechanism by which homocysteine promotes CVD is currently an active area of investigation. A recent meta-analysis that combined 3 prospective, 6 population-based, and 13 case-control studies with 5 cross-sectional studies found that elevated homocysteine was an independent, graded risk factor for arteriosclerotic vascular disease similar in magnitude to elevated serum cholesterol (Boushey, Beresford et al. 1995). The summary estimate for the odds ratio for coronary heart disease was 1.7 (95% CI, 1.5–1.9) for every 5 μmol/L increase in homocysteine, and the data raised the possibility of a stronger relationship for women. The summary estimate for cerebrovascular disease was an increased risk of 1.5 (95% CI, 1.3–1.9) for every 5 μmol/L increase. A meta-analysis of randomized controlled trials, which included the 4 previously reported large trials and 8 smaller trials, reported that folic acid supplementation did not reduce risk of CVD or all-cause mortality in individuals with pre-existing vascular or kidney disease (Bazzano, Reynolds et al. 2006). The summary relative risk (RR) for CHD was 1.04 (95% CI, 0.92–1.17) and for stroke was 0.86 (95% CI, 0.71–1.04). When these results were updated with the recent results of the Homocysteinemia in Kidney and End Stage Renal Disease (HOST) trial, then the overall OR per each 3 μmol/L reduction in tHcy levels for a mean duration of treatment of 3.1 years is 1.00 (95% CI, 0.92–1.09) for CHD events (in 12 trials) and 0.88 (95% CI, 0.78–1.00) for stroke (in 9 trials) (Baigent and Clarke 2007). A recent meta-analysis in which the efficacy of folic acid supplementation in stroke was specifically assessed has shown that lowering tHcy with folic acid may actually reduce risk of stroke by 18% (0%–32%, p = 0.045), and that the beneficial effect was greater (23%–29%) in those trials with a longer treatment duration (>36 months), larger homocysteine-lowering effects (>20%), no or partial grain fortification, and no history of stroke (Wang, Qin et al. 2007). Although this meta-analysis only included 8 trials, their conclusions are strengthened by their sensitivity analyses showing that no individual study findings influenced the overall results. Overall, results from previous randomized clinical trials assessing the efficacy of folate in combination with vitamin B_6 and/or B_{12} supplementation on the risk of CVD have been null, although there was a suggestion that homocysteine-lowering treatments could have a greater protective effect in stroke risk. The current evidence does not support the routine use of homocysteine-lowering vitamin supplements for the prevention of CVD events among individuals at high risk for vascular disease. Several ongoing large randomized trials will provide further clarity on this issue.

Homocysteine and type 2 diabetes

Although few studies have directly examined the relation between homocysteine and risk of type 2 DM, recent in vivo and in vitro studies suggest that hyperinsulinemia affects homocysteine metabolism possibly through an increased flux in the hepatic trans-sulfuration pathway (Fonseca, Mudaliar et al. 1998; House, Jacobs et al. 1999). Plasma homocysteine concentrations have been observed to be higher among obese individuals, those who are insulin resistant, and those with type 2 DM (Araki, Sako et al. 1993; Fonseca, Mudaliar et al. 1998; Das, Reynolds et al. 1999; Passaro, D'Elia et al. 2000). Changes in circulating and tissue concentrations of folic acid, vitamin B_6, and/or vitamin B_{12} have also been reported in diabetic animals and humans (Davis, Calder et al. 1976; Hargrove, Trotter et al. 1989; Araki, Sako et al. 1993; Robillon, Canivet et al. 1994). In a case-control study of 518 diabetic subjects and 371 healthy controls, serum vitamin B_6 levels were significantly lower in the diabetic subjects, with 25% having levels below the lower limit of the normal range, suggesting that people with diabetes may have an increased demand for vitamin B_6 (Davis, Calder et al. 1976). Among individuals with type 2 DM, hyperhomocysteinemia increases the risk of macrovascular complications (Munshi, Stone et al. 1996; Fonseca, Stone et al. 1997; Fonseca, Mudaliar et al. 1998). In a five-year prospective study of 2484 Dutch adults aged 50–75, hyperhomocysteinemia increased the risk for CVD death by 56% after adjustment for known CVD risk factors. For each 5 μmol/L increment of serum homocysteine, the odds ratio was 1.17 among individuals without type 2 DM and 1.60 among those with type 2 DM (Hoogeveen, Kostense et al. 2000). Munshi et al. performed methionine-load tests in 18 healthy controls, 11 diabetics without vascular disease, and 17 diabetics with vascular disease and reported that hyperhomocysteinemia occurred with significantly greater frequency (39%) in type 2 DM individuals as compared with age-matched controls (7%) (Munshi, Stone et al. 1996). The area under the curve over 24 hours, reflecting the total period of exposure to hyperhomocysteinemia, was elevated with greater frequency in individuals with type 2 DM and macrovascular disease (33%) as compared with controls (0%). Fonseca et al. measured plasma homocysteine concentrations in the fasting state and during a hyperinsulinemic-euglycemic clamp in apparently healthy subjects and in individuals with type 2 DM. Plasma homocysteine was found to decrease significantly in healthy subjects as compared to individuals with type 2 DM (from 7.2 to 6.0 mmol/L, P <.01) (Fonseca, Mudaliar et al. 1998).

While relatively few studies directly link homocysteine to the occurrence of type 2 DM, strong evidence indicates direct relations between homocysteine and vascular disease, as well as between homocysteine and lipid and hemodynamic risk factors for vascular disease. As discussed above, tissue resistance to the action of insulin has been hypothesized to be a common antecedent to both type 2 DM and atherosclerosis (Pyorala 1979; Stout 1990; Stern 1995; Pinkney, Stehouwer et al. 1997). Exposure of endothelial cells to homocysteine increases production of superoxide anion radicals and hydrogen peroxide, leading to inactivation of nitric oxide and endothelial dysfunction (Cooke and Tsao 1993; Loscalzo 1996). These data, along with the growing recognition that type 2 DM is fundamentally a vascular disease that may share common causes with CVD, strongly suggest that reducing plasma levels of homocysteine with increased intake of folic acid/vitamin B_6/vitamin B_{12} represents one promising prophylactic approach to lowering the risk of type 2 DM.

However, few human data are currently available on the relation between homocysteine levels and the risk of developing type 2 DM. In observational studies, homocysteine levels in nondiabetic individuals have been positively correlated with several biomarkers of insulin resistance and/or glucose intolerance in some (Meigs, Jacques et al. 2001; Fonseca, Fink et al. 2003; Hajer, van der Graaf et al. 2007) but not all studies (Abbasi, Facchini et al. 1999; Sheu, Lee et al. 2000; Godsland, Rosankiewicz et al. 2001). In a 4-year prospective cohort study, elevated levels of homocysteine were independently associated with a 3.6-fold increased risk of type 2 DM among 170 women with a history of gestational DM (Cho, Lim et al. 2005). These observations not only provided suggestive evidence linking elevated levels of homocysteine to the development of type 2 DM but also led to the suggestion that lowering homocysteine levels may prevent or reduce the risk of type 2 DM. If elevated homocysteine does indeed have a causal association with insulin resistance and type 2 DM, then both homocysteine-lowering agents and those with antioxidant properties could reduce the risk of type 2 DM. Dietary folic acid and vitamins B6 and B12 are the most important modifiable determinants of homocysteine levels, and adequate intake of B vitamins may be potentially beneficial for prevention of type 2 DM. This may be especially true among individuals with cardiovascular risk factors or with previous cardiovascular disease. However, no previous prospective cohort studies have specifically examined intakes of individual B vitamins and diabetes risk. Some small and short-term randomized trials for secondary prevention of diabetic complications have been conducted but yielded inconsistent results; some reported that folic acid supplementation (5–10 mg per day) reduced oxidative stress and improved endothelial function in diabetic patients during a period of 2 to 12 weeks (van Etten, de Koning et al. 2002; Hunter-Lavin, Hudson et al. 2004; Mangoni, Sherwood et al. 2005; Title, Ur et al. 2006). In a large CVD prevention trial, the Women's Antioxidant and Folic Acid Cardiovascular Study (WAFACS), daily supplementation with folic acid, vitamin B6, and vitamin B12 for 7.3 years had no significant effect on risk of type 2 DM among 4,252 women at high risk for CVD (Song, Cook et al. 2009). The WAFACS is a randomized trial of just such women, all with, or at high risk of, cardiovascular disease, who thus appear to be at increased risk of type 2 DM due to shared risk factors between the two diseases. Despite significant lowering of homocysteine levels by the combined B vitamin supplementation (18.5%), homocysteine-lowering treatment was not associated with protection against the development of type 2 DM in this randomized trial. It is unknown whether a greater magnitude of homocysteine-lowering would have conferred protection against diabetes.

Vitamin D

Vitamin D biology and deficiency

Vitamin D3 (cholecalciferol) is the natural form of vitamin D that has been widely used as a supplement (Norman 2008). Vitamin D3 is produced in the skin by an ultraviolet light-induced photolytic conversion of 7-dehy-drocholesterol to previtamin D3 followed by thermal isomerization to vitamin D3 (Norman 2008). Vitamin D is obtained as vitamin D2 or D3 from diet, supplements, or D3 from conversion of 7-dehydrocholesterol in the skin by ultraviolet B radiation, and is hydroxylated in the liver to 25-hydroxyvitamin D [25(OH)D], the major circulating vitamin D metabolite (Dawson-Hughes, Heaney et al. 2005; Giovannucci 2005). 25(OH) D is further synthesized by 1α-hydroxylase to 1,25-dihydroxyvitamin D [1,25(OH)$_2$D]. Only the 1,25(OH)$_2$D3 is a metabolically active form of vitamin D (Holick 2007; Norman 2008). Vitamin D is well known for its essential role in calcium homeostasis and bone metabolism. However, a large body of evidence from both observational and experimental studies has clearly suggested its other physiologic effects, especially those on individual or combined metabolic parameters such as adiposity, blood pressure, lipid metabolism, glucose intolerance, insulin secretion, and the metabolic syndrome (Norman, Frankel et al. 1980; Boucher 1998; Holick 2004; Mathieu, Gysemans et al. 2005; Davis and Dwyer 2007; Holick 2007; Pittas, Lau et al. 2007; Norman 2008; Palomer, Gonzalez-Clemente et al. 2008; Penckofer, Kouba et al. 2008; Giovannucci 2009). Emerging evidence has linked low vitamin D levels to the pathogenesis of diabetes and its complications (Mathieu, Gysemans et al. 2005; Pittas, Lau et al. 2007; Palomer, Gonzalez-Clemente et al. 2008).

Vitamin D deficiency is a common public health problem nationwide (Holick 2004). It has been associated with many adverse health outcomes, including several bone diseases, certain types of cancer, multiple autoimmune diseases, and the metabolic syndrome (Holick 2004; Dawson-Hughes, Heaney et al. 2005; Giovannucci 2005; Pittas, Lau et al. 2007). Circulating 25(OH)D, which reflects all sources of vitamin D exposure and has a half-life of 2–3 weeks, has been widely used as a reliable surrogate of vitamin D status (Holick 2007; Norman 2008). Due to differences in assay methods and population characteristics, there is no consensus on the cutoff values defining vitamin D insufficiency or deficiency. However, vitamin D insufficiency has been previously reported to range from levels of 40 to 75 nmol/L (16 to 30 ng/mL), and vitamin D deficiency is generally defined as levels of <50 nmol/L (20 ng/mL) (Malabanan, Veronikis et al. 1998; Bischoff-Ferrari, Giovannucci et al. 2006; Holick 2007). Vitamin D deficiency is likely determined by many factors such as age, sex, race/skin pigmentation, season, geographic latitude, food and supplemental sources of vitamin D, adiposity, and genetic predisposition. In particular, low vitamin D status among the elderly is a potential public health problem. Several studies have found a high prevalence of vitamin D deficiency among older individuals (Gloth, Gundberg et al. 1995; LeBoff, Kohlmeier et al. 1999). Aging may decrease the ability of skin to produce the necessary precursors for vitamin D synthesis (MacLaughlin and Holick 1985). Also, the elderly may increase their risk of vitamin D deficiency by lack of sun exposure or consuming a diet poor in vitamin D.

Vitamin D and insulin secretion and sensitivity

A large body of literature has suggested that optimal vitamin D homeostasis is essential for both insulin action and secretion (Norman, Frankel et al. 1980; Boucher 1998; Mathieu, Gysemans et al. 2005; Davis and Dwyer 2007; Holick 2007; Pittas, Lau et al. 2007; Norman 2008; Palomer, Gonzalez-Clemente et al. 2008; Penckofer, Kouba et al. 2008; Tai, Need et al. 2008; Giovannucci 2009), which are two fundamental features in the pathogenesis of T2D. Vitamin D may directly affect pancreatic β-cell function by the binding of circulating 1,25-dihydroxyvitamin D to the VDR in β-cells (Figure 5.3) (Norman, Frankel et al. 1980; Cade and Norman 1986). In vitro

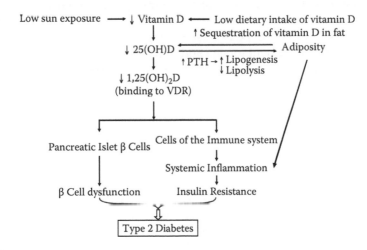

Figure 5.3 Hypothesized mechanisms underlying the relation between vitamin D deficiency and type 2 diabetes.

studies clearly show impaired insulin secretion from islets of vitamin D-deficient rats (Norman, Frankel et al. 1980; Kadowaki and Norman 1984; Billaudel, Faure et al. 1989). Genetically disrupted VDR gene in mice led to a pronounced impairment in insulin secretory capacity with a reduction in pancreatic insulin mRNA levels (Zeitz, Weber et al. 2003), while maintaining normal pancreatic islet mass, architecture, and islet neogenesis. Vitamin D may also indirectly affect calcium-dependent insulin secretion via regulation of calcium transport through the β-cells (Milner and Hales 1967; Beaulieu, Kestekian et al. 1993). Intravenous administration of 1,25(OH)D3 increased insulin secretion and reduced blood glucose excursion in response to an intravenous glucose load in vitamin D-deficient rats (Cade and Norman 1986) and rabbits (Nyomba, Bouillon et al. 1984). The effect of vitamin D on insulin resistance may not be direct and could be through beneficial effects on adiposity. Several other mechanisms, including stimulating expression of insulin receptors, regulation of the calcium pool, and modulation of cytokine expression and activity, may also account for improvement of insulin action in peripheral tissues (Holick 2007; Norman 2008).

Human data also support the hypothesis that low vitamin D status is associated with impaired β-cell function, insulin resistance, and impaired glucose intolerance (Figure 5.4). Many cross-sectional studies among nondiabetic individuals have specifically examined the associations of dietary or serum vitamin D levels with surrogate biomarkers of glucose homeostasis such as hemoglobin A1c (HbA1c), and HOMA-IR and HOMA-B (Need, Morris et al. 1993; Scragg, Holdaway et al. 1995; Snijder, van Dam et al. 2005). For example, a recent cross-sectional study of 808 nondiabetic participants of the Framingham Offspring Study has reported an association between plasma 25(OH)D and markers of the insulin-resistant phenotype assessed using 2h 75 g OGTT (Liu, Meigs et al. 2009). After adjustment for age and sex, plasma 25(OH)D was positively associated with insulin sensitivity index, but this association was no longer significant after further adjustment for BMI, waist circumference, and current smoking status. 25(OH)D remained inversely associated with fasting plasma glucose (lowest tertile vs. highest tertile: –1.6%; p for trend = 0.007), fasting plasma insulin (–9.8%; p for trend = 0.001), and lower HOMA-IR score (–12.7%; p for trend < 0.001) (Liu, Meigs et al. 2009). Some cross-sectional studies provided correlations with more accurate assessments of insulin sensitivity and/or secretion such as the hyperinsulinemic-euglycemic clamp. For example, among 126 healthy, glucose-tolerant individuals living in California, 25(OH)D levels were positively associated with insulin sensitivity ($r = 0.46$, $P < 0.0001$) and inversely associated with first-phase insulin response ($r = -0.25$, $P = 0.0045$) and second-phase insulin response ($r = -0.35$, $P = 0.0001$) as measured by the hyperglycemic clamp (Chiu, Chu et al. 2004). In addition, it is biologically plausible that the link between vitamin D and insulin resistance may simply reflect the detrimental effects of proinflammatory cytokines produced by adipose tissue (such as TNF-α and IL-6) on insulin resistance or glucose uptake (Mohamed-Ali, Pinkney et al. 1998; Wajchenberg 2000; Kershaw and Flier 2004).

Few human studies have examined the effects of vitamin D supplementation on glucose homeostasis and insulin resistance among individuals without clinical diabetes (Gedik and Akalin 1986; Boucher, Mannan et al. 1995; Fliser, Stefanski et al. 1997; Pittas, Harris et al. 2007; Nagpal, Pande et al. 2009). Earlier small and nonrandomized open-label trials provided support for the potential beneficial effects of vitamin D treatment on insulin secretion and sensitivity (Boucher, Mannan et al. 1995; Gedik and Akalin 1986). Given the sample sizes and short duration, these clinical trials did not have adequate power to address this issue. Furthermore, differences in study population and intervention periods, coupled with the fact that different vitamin D doses and forms were used, may explain the variable findings from these previous trials. In a randomized, placebo-controlled trial of 1,25-(OH)2D3 treatment (1.5 ug/day for 7 days) in 18 healthy white males, vitamin D treatment did not change mean glucose, insulin, or insulin sensitivity (Fliser, Stefanski et al. 1997). However, recent evidence from a large randomized trial with a long follow-up period appeared to support the causal effect of vitamin D supplementation on insulin sensitivity, at least in older adults with impaired glucose tolerance (Pittas, Harris et al. 2007). In this trial of 314 adults aged 65 years and older, taking a combined vitamin D and calcium supplement (700 IU vitamin D3 and 500 mg calcium) for 3 years prevented increases in fasting plasma glucose and insulin resistance (measured by HOMA-IR) among glucose-intolerant participants (Pittas, Harris et al. 2007).

Observational evidence for vitamin D and type 2 DM

Numerous clinical and epidemiologic studies have investigated the association of serum and dietary vitamin D with type 2 DM in humans. Some cross-sectional studies have reported inverse associations between dietary vitamin D and diabetes risk factors, including decreased insulin secretion, glucose intolerance, insulin resistance, as well as the prevalence of the metabolic syndrome. Most relevant observational studies using dietary assessment information focused on vitamin-D-rich food groups such as dairy products and fish rather than specifically examined dietary intake of vitamin D (Choi, Willett et al. 2005; Liu, Choi et al. 2006; Elwood, Pickering et al. 2007; Snijder, van der Heijden et al. 2007). In the Women's Health Study of 10,066 apparently healthy and nondiabetic participants, there was an inverse association between total and dietary vitamin D and the prevalence of metabolic syndrome (OR for highest versus the lowest quartiles of dietary vitamin D = 0.85, 95% CI, 0.70–1.02) (Liu, Song et al. 2005). One large prospective study has reported the relation between dietary vitamin D intake and subsequent diabetes risk. In the Nurses' Health Study of 83,779 women, total and dietary vitamin D intakes were inversely associated with risk of type 2 diabetes over a 20-year follow-up period (RR for highest versus the lowest quartiles of dietary vitamin D = 0.81, 95% CI, 0.64 to 1.01) (Pittas, Dawson-Hughes et al. 2006). It should be noted that dietary vitamin D intake is likely flawed by measurement error and also does not reflect the major nondietary component of vitamin D from sun exposure. The observed associations of dietary vitamin D intake with improved glucose metabolism and decreased risk of incident diabetes may be the results of confounding or of other components of foods that are highly correlated with vitamin D and calcium. In fact, the nonsignificant results also reflect the fact that dietary vitamin D, compared with endogenous 7-dehydrocholesterol conversion, is not the major source of vitamin D in the body.

Circulating 25(OH)D, which reflects all sources of vitamin D exposure and has a half-life of 2–3 weeks, is a comprehensive and stable indicator of vitamin D status (Hollis and Napoli 1985; Hollis, Kamerud et al. 1993; Holick 2007). Epidemiological evidence relating lower circulating vitamin D levels to hyperglycemia, insulin resistance, or prevalent type 2 DM primarily derives from cross-sectional reports (Scragg, Sowers et al. 2004; Ford, Ajani et al. 2005; Need, O'Loughlin et al. 2005; Hypponen, Boucher et al. 2008). Prospective data are relatively limited. Recently, one prospective study of 524 nondiabetic individuals aged 40–69 years reported inverse associations between baseline serum 25(OH)D and the incidences of hyperglycemia, insulin resistance, and the metabolic syndrome after 10 years of follow-up (Forouhi, Luan et al. 2008). In the adjusted models controlling for age, sex, smoking, BMI, physical activity, social class, season, and baseline levels of parathyroid hormone (PTH) and calcium, each 25 nmol/L increase in serum 25(OH)D at baseline (which is equivalent to 1 SD of the 25(OH)D distribution in this population) was significantly associated with a decrease in 10-year follow-up of fasting glucose (–0.05 mmol/L), 2-h glucose (–0.25 mmol/L), fasting insulin (4.2 pmol/L), in HOMA-IR (–0.16 units), and metabolic syndrome risk (–0.05 unit z score) (Forouhi, Luan et al. 2008). The relationship between baseline circulating 25(OH)D and type 2 DM incidence has been assessed among Finnish populations in one small cohort study and two nested case-control reports, and all showed an inverse association (Mattila, Knekt et al. 2007; Knekt, Laaksonen et al. 2008). In the Mini-Finland Health Survey, with 187 incident type 2 DM cases among 4,097 participants aged 40–69 followed for 17 years, a statistically significant inverse association was observed between serum 25(OH)D concentration and incidence of type 2 DM (RR comparing the highest [71 nmol/L] to lowest quartile [22 nmol/L]: 0.60, 95% CI,

0.36–0.98; p for trend = 0.01) (Mattila, Knekt et al. 2007). However, this association was attenuated after further adjustments for BMI, leisure-time exercise, smoking, and education (RR, 0.70; 95% CI, 0.42–1.16; p for trend = 0.07) (Mattila, Knekt et al. 2007). Most recently, a pooled analysis of two nested case-control studies of 412 incident type 2 DM cases and 986 controls with 22 years of follow-up found an even stronger inverse association in men, but not among women, after adjustment for confounding factors (the highest [69 nmol/L] vs. lowest quartile [22 nmol/L]: OR = 0.28 [0.10-0.81] in men and 1.14 [0.60–2.17] in women) (Knekt, Laaksonen et al. 2008). The reason for the sex difference is unclear but may result from residual confounding and statistical fluctuation due to the small sample size. Due to possible confounding effects, prospective data on serum 25(OH)D and type 2 DM have been suggestive and inconclusive.

Additional support for the hypothesis originates from genetic association studies that reported a link between VDR polymorphisms and obesity, insulin sensitivity, insulin secretion, and T2D (Ye, Reis et al. 2001; Ogunkolade, Boucher et al. 2002; Oh and Barrett-Connor 2002; Ortlepp, Metrikat et al. 2003). Such genetic research is useful to better our understanding of the role of vitamin D and VDR in the development of chronic metabolic disorders, as the pleiotropic properties of vitamin D are mainly mediated through its receptor (Holick 2007; Norman 2008; Sone, Marx et al. 1990; Fang, van Meurs et al. 2005). Despite some intriguing findings, in the aggregate, population genetic association data have focused on VDR and provided little or no conclusive evidence (Ye, Reis et al. 2001; Ogunkolade, Boucher et al. 2002; Oh and Barrett-Connor 2002; Malecki, Frey et al. 2003; Ortlepp, Metrikat et al. 2003). Further studies integrating genetic variants of all relevant genes in the vitamin D metabolism pathway with circulating 25(OH)D will better characterize the relation of vitamin D to type 2 DM risk and provide new insight into the effects of vitamin D.

Randomized trials of vitamin D and diabetes-related endpoints

Data from randomized clinical trials, albeit limited, suggest a protective effect of vitamin D treatment on insulin secretion and action in both nondiabetic and diabetic patients. Some but not all trials have observed beneficial effects on insulin secretion, glucose homeostasis, and insulin resistance. These trials are limited by design due to small sample sizes, short intervention periods, nonrandomized treatment allocation, and the lack of objective assessment of vitamin D status and insulin or glucose homeostasis.

In a randomized, placebo-controlled trial of 35 patients with T2D, 1,25 dihydroxyvitamin D3 [1,25-(OH) 2D3] treatment (1 μg/day for 4 days) had no effect on fasting insulin or glucose levels (Orwoll, Riddle et al. 1994). However, those with a shorter duration of diabetes showed a greater improvement in insulin secretion, indicating that vitamin D may exert effects earlier in the progression of diabetes (Orwoll, Riddle et al. 1994). In another randomized, placebo-controlled trial of 1,25-(OH)2D3 treatment (1.5 µg/day for 7 days) in 18 healthy white men, vitamin D treatment did not change mean glucose, insulin, or insulin sensitivity (Fliser, Stefanski et al. 1997). Given the sample sizes and short duration, these clinical trials did not have adequate power. Recent evidence from three relatively large randomized trials provided additional data on the causal effect of vitamin D supplementation on glucose tolerance and insulin action/secretion (Pittas, Harris et al. 2007; Nagpal, Pande et al. 2009; Zittermann, Frisch et al. 2009). In a randomized trial of 100 apparently healthy, middle-aged, centrally obese men, short-term oral supplementation with vitamin D3 (120,000 IU per 2 weeks) for 6 weeks resulted in significantly increased postprandial insulin sensitivity index assessed by 3h OGTT ($P = 0.038$ for mean difference), whereas other secondary insulin sensitivity or secretion indices were unaltered (Nagpal, Pande et al. 2009). Also, among 300 healthy overweight participants (with mean 25[OH]D levels of 12 ng/ml), a 1-year randomized trial of vitamin D treatment (83 µg/day) did not change HbA1c levels and fasting levels of glucose and proinsulin but significantly reduced levels of tumor necrosis factor-α (TNF-α) (–10.2% in the vitamin D group compared with –3.2% in the placebo group, $P = 0.049$) (Zittermann, Frisch et al. 2009). Pittas et al. conducted a relatively large trial of 314 adults aged 65 years and older with 3 years of treatment duration (Pittas, Harris et al. 2007). Combined vitamin D and calcium supplementation (700 IU vitamin D3 and 500 mg calcium) prevented increases in fasting plasma glucose ($P = 0.042$) and insulin resistance (measured by HOMA-IR) ($P = 0.031$) among impaired glucose-tolerant participants but not among those with normal fasting glucose (Pittas, Harris et al. 2007). It is noteworthy that differences in study population, intervention periods, metabolic profiles, and vitamin D status, coupled with the fact that different vitamin D doses and forms were used, may explain the inconsistent results from these previous trials.

The largest randomized trial, the Women's Health Initiative Clinical Trial, has to date evaluated vitamin D supplementation for the primary prevention of type 2 DM. This large trial of 33,951 initially nondiabetic postmenopausal women did not observe any effect from daily intake of 1,000 mg elemental calcium plus 400 IU vitamin D3 on the risk of incident diabetes over 7 years of follow-up (de Boer, Tinker et al. 2008). However, the dose of 400 IU vitamin D3 daily may have been too low to impart a clinical benefit. In particular, median levels of serum 25(OH)D were raised from 42.3 to 54.1 nmol/L (roughly 12 nmol/L), which is lower than the optimal value of 90 nmol/L or more for its role in skeletal and nonskeletal health, including type 2 DM (Dawson-Hughes, Heaney et al. 2005). Hence, there is a need for large-scale clinical trials of high-dose vitamin D supplementation to clarify the beneficial effects of vitamin

D supplementation on primary prevention of type 2 DM. A large-scale VITamin D and OmegA-3 TriaL (VITAL), a randomized trial of supplemental vitamin D (2000 IU/d) and marine omega-3 fatty acids, is currently under way for the primary prevention of CVD and cancer. Several ancillary studies within the VITAL cohort are also being conducted to address the balance of benefits and risks of vitamin D supplementation for other chronic diseases, including type 2 DM, hypertension, autoimmune disease, chronic lung disease. Evidence from randomized trials such as VITAL is critical for establishing cause-and-effect relationships between vitamin D and health outcomes.

Magnesium

Magnesium intake and deficiency

Magnesium is an essential mineral with several dietary sources including whole grains, green leafy vegetables, legumes, and nuts (Groff and Gropper 2000; Cleveland, Goldman et al. 1994; Vaquero 2002). National survey data indicate that dietary magnesium intake is inadequate in the US general population, particularly among adolescent girls, adult women, and the elderly (Vaquero 2002; Ford and Mokdad 2003). Magnesium content tends to be lost substantially during the refining and processing of foods. A survey in a nationally representative sample of US adults indicates that the average magnesium intake in the United States is below the Daily Reference Intakes, particularly among adolescent females, adult females, and the elderly (Pennington and Young 1991; Cleveland, Goldman et al. 1994; Vaquero 2002; Ford and Mokdad 2003). Magnesium status in the human body is a result of interactions among dietary intake, intestinal absorption, renal excretion, and exchange from bone (Saris, Mervaala et al. 2000). Homeostasis of magnesium is tightly regulated and depends on the balance between intestinal absorption and renal excretion. Emerging evidence has indicated a genetic basis for magnesium metabolism in humans. Because magnesium content is low in diets high in meats and dairy products and tends to be lost substantially during the refining and processing of foods, the adoption of a "Western diet" characterized by high intakes of red and processed meat as well as other components, including diary products and other highly refined or prepared foods, is believed to contribute to suboptimal intake of magnesium in the general population of industrialized countries (Groff and Gropper 2000; Cleveland, Goldman et al. 1994; Vaquero 2002). Adequate magnesium intake is believed to be important in maintaining the magnesium status in the human body (Saris, Mervaala et al. 2000).

Abdominal obesity and insulin resistance

Obesity, particularly abdominal or visceral adiposity, has consistently been demonstrated as a fundamental cause of insulin resistance and type 2 DM (Wilson and Kannel 2002; Wilson and Grundy 2003). Some epidemiologic studies have examined directly the effects of whole grains on body weight and weight changes (Liu, Willett et al. 2003; Koh-Banerjee, Franz et al. 2004; McKeown, Meigs et al. 2004). The observed associations between improved insulin sensitivity and components in whole grains including magnesium have been attributed, at least in part, to the beneficial effects of whole grains on body weight or weight changes. However, few studies have specifically examined the direct effect of magnesium intake on body weight.

Magnesium may play a role in glucose homeostasis, insulin action in peripheral tissues, and pancreatic insulin secretion (Saris, Mervaala et al. 2000; Barbagallo, Dominguez et al. 2003). Although the exact mechanisms are not well understood, several mechanisms have been proposed. First, magnesium functions as a cofactor for several enzymes critical for glucose metabolism utilizing high-energy phosphate bonds (Saris, Mervaala et al. 2000). Diminished levels of magnesium were observed to decrease tyrosine kinase activity at insulin receptors (Suarez, Pulido et al. 1995) and to increase intracellular calcium levels (Barbagallo, Dominguez et al. 2003), leading to an impairment in insulin signaling. Thus, intracellular magnesium levels have been hypothesized to be important for maintaining insulin sensitivity in skeletal muscle or adipose tissue (Paolisso and Barbagallo 1997; Barbagallo, Dominguez et al. 2003). Additionally, intracellular magnesium levels may also influence glucose-stimulated insulin secretion in pancreatic β-cells through altered cellular ion metabolism (Barbagallo, Dominguez et al. 2003), oxidative stress (Giugliano, Paolisso et al. 1996), and the proinflammatory response (Weglicki, Phillips et al. 1992; Kurantsin-Mills, Cassidy et al. 1997).

Epidemiologic evidence suggests an important role of magnesium in insulin sensitivity. Some cross-sectional studies have shown an inverse association between plasma or erythrocyte magnesium levels and fasting insulin levels in both diabetic patients and apparently healthy individuals (Ma, Folsom et al. 1995; Rosolova, Mayer et al. 2000). Several epidemiologic studies have also found an association between dietary magnesium intake and insulin homeostasis quantified by insulin the clamp technique (Humphries, Kushner et al. 1999). Similarly, a significant inverse association between dietary magnesium intake and fasting insulin concentrations was observed in several population-based cross-sectional studies (Manolio, Savage et al. 1991; Ma, Folsom et al. 1995; Fung, Manson et al. 2003; Song, Manson et al. 2004). However, as in any cross-sectional studies, the observed associations cannot be established as causal.

Several short-term metabolic studies and small randomized trials have specifically examined the efficacy of magnesium supplementation in improving insulin sensitivity among nondiabetic individuals, but the results have varied. Rosolova et al. have reported a relationship between plasma magnesium concentration and insulin-mediated glucose disposal (Rosolova, Mayer et al. 1997, 2000). In a study of 18 nondiabetic partici-pants, those with low levels of fasting plasma magnesium (<0.80 mmol/L) had significantly higher plasma glucose and insulin concentrations after a 75-g oral glucose tolerance test (OGTT) and were more resistant to insu-lin-mediated glucose disposal reflected by higher steady-state plasma glu-cose concentrations after a modification of insulin suppression test than those with high levels of plasma magnesium (>0.83 mmol/L) (Rosolova, Mayer et al. 1997). Both groups were comparable in terms of sex, family history of diabetes, history of hypertension, cigarette smoking, alcohol consumption, and steady-state insulin concentrations. Similar associa-tions between plasma magnesium concentrations and insulin-mediated glucose disposal were also observed when the same investigators enrolled 98 healthy nondiabetic individuals (Rosolova, Mayer et al. 2000). One non-randomized trial examined the effect of magnesium supplementation on insulin sensitivity in 12 nondiabetic participants with normal body weight (Nadler, Buchanan et al. 1993). A magnesium-deficient diet (<0.5 mmol/day) for 4 weeks led to approximately 25% reduction in an insulin sensitivity index determined by minimal model analysis using a modi-fied intravenous glucose tolerance test (Nadler, Buchanan et al. 1993). Two randomized double-blind placebo-controlled trials have also assessed the effects of magnesium in both insulin secretion and action among non-diabetic participants (Paolisso, Sgambato et al. 1992; Guerrero-Romero, Tamez-Perez et al. 2004). In one trial of 12 nonobese elderly participants, daily magnesium supplementation (4.5 g magnesium pidolate, equivalent to 15.8 mmol) for 4 weeks significantly improved glucose-induced insulin response and insulin-mediated glucose disposal (Paolisso, Sgambato et al. 1992). In another randomized double-blind placebo-controlled trial, 60 apparently healthy participants who had low serum magnesium concen-trations and insulin resistance assessed by the homeostasis model analy-sis for insulin resistance (HOMA-IR) were randomly allocated to receive either magnesium supplement (2.5 g/day magnesium chloride [12.5 mmol elemental magnesium]) or placebo (Guerrero-Romero, Tamez-Perez et al. 2004). Magnesium treatment for 3 months significantly improved insulin resistance as reflected by fasting glucose (5.8 ± 0.9 to 5.0 ± 0.6 mmol/L), insulin (103.2 ± 56.4 to 70.2 ± 29.6 mmol/L), and HOMA-IR (4.6 ± 2.8 to 2.6 ± 1.1, P < 0.0001) (Guerrero-Romero, Tamez-Perez et al. 2004). Due to limited evidence, the beneficial effect of magnesium supplementation in improv-ing insulin sensitivity in nondiabetic people has yet to be conclusively demonstrated, and future long-term and well-designed controlled trials are warranted.

Epidemiologic evidence provides further support for an important role of magnesium in insulin sensitivity. Some cross-sectional studies have shown an inverse association between plasma or erythrocyte magnesium levels and fasting insulin levels in both diabetic patients and apparently healthy individuals (Ma, Folsom et al. 1995; Rosolova, Mayer et al. 2000). Several epidemiologic studies have also found an association between dietary magnesium intake and insulin homeostasis (Manolio, Savage et al. 1991; Ma, Folsom et al. 1995; Fung, Manson et al. 2003; Song, Manson et al. 2004). Several short-term metabolic studies and small randomized trials have also specifically examined the efficacy of magnesium supplementation in improving insulin sensitivity among nondiabetic individuals, although the evidence remains inconclusive (Nadler, Buchanan et al. 1993; Paolisso, Sgambato et al. 1992; Guerrero-Romero, Tamez-Perez et al. 2004). Specifically, two randomized double-blind placebo-controlled trials found that magnesium supplementation improved both insulin secretion and insulin action among nondiabetic participants (Paolisso, Sgambato et al. 1992; Guerrero-Romero, Tamez-Perez et al. 2004).

Dyslipidemia

Dietary magnesium may also be related to lipid metabolism independent of its effects on insulin sensitivity. As a cofactor for many rate-limiting enzymes critical for lipid metabolism, magnesium may decrease the activity of lecithin:cholesterol acyl-transferase (LCAT) (Itoh, Kawasaka et al. 1997) and the HMG-CoA reductase, and increase lipoprotein lipase activity (Rayssiguier, Noe et al. 1991). LCAT is an enzyme that esterifies free cholesterol, which lowers LDL cholesterol (LDL-C) and triglyceride levels and raises HDL cholesterol (HDL-C) levels. HMG-CoA reductase is a rate-limiting enzyme in cholesterol biosynthesis. The lipoprotein lipase is responsible for the conversion of triglycerides to HDL-C and thus leads to a decrease in hepatic VLDL-triglyceride synthesis and secretion. Animal studies have shown favorable effects of magnesium intake on lipid metabolism by lowering serum cholesterol and triglycerides (Vitale, White et al. 1957; Rayssiguier, Gueux et al. 1981; Rayssiguier 1984; Altura, Brust et al. 1990).

Epidemiologic evidence, predominantly from cross-sectional studies, suggests a role for magnesium in improving blood lipid profiles (Guerrero-Romero and Rodriguez-Moran 2002). Several large-scale observational studies have examined the associations between dietary magnesium intake and lipid profiles and found that magnesium intake was significantly associated with high HDL-C and low triglyceride in US cohorts of women and men (Ma, Folsom et al. 1995; Song, Ridker et al. 2005; He, Liu et al. 2006). The associations also appeared to be independent of body fatness and insulin resistance. Several trials have evaluated the direct effect of magnesium supplements on blood lipids and lipoproteins among normal or hyperlipidemic patients without or with other overt chronic diseases. Four randomized, double-blind, placebo-controlled trials have evaluated the effects of oral magnesium supplementation on blood lipids and lipoproteins among nondiabetic participants. Several trials (Itoh, Kawasaka et al. 1997; Rasmussen, Aurup et al. 1989; Kirsten, Heintz et al. 1988) provided some evidence in support of the role of magnesium supplementation on improving dyslipidemia, but one did not (Marken, Weart et al. 1989). Overall, oral magnesium supplementation (7.4–15 mmol/day elemental magnesium) for 4–12 weeks was reported to significantly increase HDL-C (6%–7%), triglycerides (3%), and apolipoprotein (apo) A1 (2%) and decrease serum LDL-C concentrations (8%) and apo B (15%) (Itoh, Kawasaka et al. 1997; Rasmussen, Aurup et al. 1989; Kirsten, Heintz et al. 1988). For diabetic patients, more than 20 human metabolic studies and clinical trials have yielded apparently conflicting results (Karppanen, Tanskanen et al. 1984; Sjogren, Floren et al. 1988; Paolisso, Sgambato et al. 1989; Gullestad, Jacobsen et al. 1994; Paolisso, Scheen et al. 1994; Purvis, Cummings et al. 1994; Eibl, Kopp et al. 1995; Eriksson and Kohvakka 1995; de Lourdes Lima, Cruz et al. 1998; de Valk, Verkaaik et al. 1998; Rodriguez-Moran and Guerrero-Romero 2003; Yokota, Kato et al. 2004). A meta-analysis of all randomized double-blinded controlled trials (n = 9) showed that oral magnesium supplementation (median = 15 mmol/day or 360 mg/day) for 4–16 weeks appeared to increase HDL-C levels (0.08 mmol/L, 95% CI, 0.03–0.14 mmol/L) among a total of 370 patients with type 2 DM; however, it caused no significant changes in total cholesterol, LDL-C, or triglycerides. It is noteworthy that the effect of magnesium supplementation seemed to be most pronounced in individuals at high risk for insulin resistance and magnesium deficiency; a randomized double-blind placebo-controlled trial of 60 apparently healthy participants reported that magnesium intake (2.5 g/day magnesium chloride [12.5 mmol]) for 3 months significantly reduced total cholesterol (10.7%) and triglycerides (39.3%) and LDL-C (11.8%) and increased HDL-C (22.2%) only among participants who had insulin resistance and low serum magnesium concentrations (Guerrero-Romero, Tamez-Perez et al. 2004). Taken together, these studies suggest that magnesium intake or supplementation raised HDL-C levels in normal people, diabetic patients, and patients with hyperlipidemia and cardiovascular disease. Because of limited data from large-scale well-designed epidemiologic studies, the relationship between magnesium intake and other lipids and lipoproteins independent of insulin resistance remains largely unknown.

Hypertension

A substantial body of research has accumulated for decades, implicating a pivotal role of magnesium intake in blood pressure (BP) regulation (Touyz 2003). In vitro studies have shown that magnesium has multiple functions that may contribute to its antihypertensive effects (Touyz 2003). The proposed underlying mechanisms include the inhibition of intracellular calcium mobilization as a calcium antagonist, attenuation of the adverse effect of sodium by stimulating activity of sodium-potassium (Na-K) ATPase or increasing urinary excretion of sodium, decreased release of catecholamine (Seelig and Heggtveit 1974; Touyz 2003), improvement of myocardial contractility and vascular smooth muscle tone (Seelig and Heggtveit 1974), endothelium-dependent vasodilation (Yamori and Mizushima 2000; Chakraborti, Chakraborti et al. 2002; Touyz 2003), systemic inflammation (Guerrero-Romero and Rodriguez-Moran 2002; Song, Ford et al. 2005), and insulin secretion and action (Paolisso and Barbagallo 1997; Barbagallo, Dominguez et al. 2003).

The hypothetical relation between magnesium intake and BP was suggested by the results from ecologic studies that showed a negative correlation between water hardness and BP and hypertension (Stitt, Clayton et al. 1973; Dawson, Frey et al. 1978). The majority of epidemiologic data relating dietary magnesium to a lower prevalence of hypertension is provided by numerous cross-sectional studies. Results from most, but not all cross-sectional studies, suggest that magnesium intake reduces BP in diverse populations (Mizushima, Cappuccio et al. 1998; Yamori and Mizushima 2000). Results from observational studies have been thoroughly reviewed elsewhere (Whelton and Klag 1989; Mizushima, Cappuccio et al. 1998). A qualitative review of 29 observational studies concluded that there was an inverse association between dietary magnesium intake and BP, which was relatively consistent across studies using different study populations and sample sizes, various methodologies of diet assessment, and different statistical analyses (Mizushima, Cappuccio et al. 1998). However, the evidence from cross-sectional studies does not necessarily imply any causal relation due to the inherent limitation of this study design.

Prospective data on the relation of magnesium intake with the development of hypertension are very limited (Witteman, Willett et al. 1989; Ascherio, Rimm et al. 1992; Peacock, Folsom et al. 1999). In the Women's Health Study, Song et al. reported that high intake of magnesium at baseline was modestly associated with a lower 10-year risk of incident hypertension among apparent healthy middle-aged and older US women (Song, Sesso et al. 2006). Similar effects were observed among those nonsmokers with no history of diabetes or high cholesterol levels who were less likely to change their diet. These data are similar to those from the Nurses' Health Study and the Health Professionals Follow-up Study, which have reported a significant inverse association between dietary magnesium intake and BP (Witteman, Willett et al. 1989; Ascherio, Rimm et al. 1992). In the Nurses' Health Study, Ascherio et al. observed an inverse relation of dietary magnesium with self-reported BP but not with the incidence of hypertension. After adjusting for age, BMI, and alcohol intake, the RR of incident hypertension was 1.10 (95% CI: 0.92–1.32; P for trend = 0.56) and the average BP was 1.3/1.0 mm Hg lower in women with high intake (≥350 mg/d) than those with low magnesium intake (<200 mg/d) (Ascherio, Hennekens et al. 1996). In contrast, the Atherosclerosis Risk in Communities (ARIC) study failed to detect a significant association between dietary magnesium and hypertension (Peacock, Folsom et al. 1999). Although the ARIC study found a modest inverse association between serum magnesium levels and incident hypertension, the correlation between serum and dietary magnesium in this study was very low (correlation coefficient = 0.053) (Peacock, Folsom et al. 1999). In the Coronary Artery Risk Development in Young Adults Study (CARDIA) with follow-up of 15 years, dietary magnesium intake was inversely associated with incident hypertension (P for trend < 0.01), but this association was substantially attenuated toward the null after adjustment for dietary factors including total energy, fiber, polyunsaturated fat, saturated fat, and total carbohydrates (He, Liu et al. 2006). The available evidence for the role of magnesium in primary prevention of hypertension is not compelling, but we cannot rule out a small effect of high magnesium intake in lowering blood pressure among normotensive people. To reconcile the discrepancies in the results from these previous prospective cohort studies, the data regarding the association between dietary magnesium intake and incidence of hypertension were pooled using a classic random-effect meta-analysis (DerSimonian and Laird 1986). A $\chi 2$ statistic was used to test between-study heterogeneity (Petitti 2000). The summary estimate of RR is 0.88 comparing the highest category of dietary magnesium intake with the lowest category of intake (95% CI: 0.80–0.97; P = 0.87 for between-study heterogeneity). Considering the partial influence shared by other highly correlated variables such as fiber, calcium, and potassium, dietary magnesium may have only a modest effect on the risk of hypertension.

Numerous small clinical trials have assessed the therapeutic effect of magnesium supplements in hypertension but yielded inconsistent results (Mizushima, Cappuccio et al. 1998; Jee, Miller et al. 2002). Many sources of heterogeneity may have contributed to the inconsistency in these trials, including small sample size, incomplete randomization, the lack of blinding in design, variable duration of follow-up, high rates of noncompliance, and differences in magnesium treatment protocols, magnesium formulation and dose, and study populations. In a recent meta-analysis of clinical trials between 1983 and 2001, Jee et al. identified 20 randomized trials with a sample size from 13 to 461 participants (median: 31 per trial) and a follow-up period from 3 to 24 weeks (median: 8.5 weeks) (Jee, Miller et al. 2002). Their results showed that magnesium supplementation led to a small overall reduction in BP in a dose-dependent manner. For each 10 mmol/day (240 mg/day) increase in magnesium dose, systolic BP decreased by 4.3 mmHg (95% CI: −6.3 to −2.2; P for trend < 0.001) and diastolic BP by 2.3 mmHg (95% CI: −4.9 to 0; P for trend = 0.09) (Jee, Miller et al. 2002). Furthermore, the pooled results of 14 double-blind randomized trials among hypertensive patients showed that a 10 mmol/day (240 mg/day) increase in magnesium intake was associated with a decrease in both systolic BP (3.3 mmHg, 95% CI: −0.1 to 6.8) and diastolic BP (2.3 mmHg, 95% CI: −1.0 to 5.6) (Jee, Miller et al. 2002). Overall, the evidence from these trials suggests a modest antihypertensive effect by magnesium supplementation, although additional research is needed to assess whether magnesium therapy is beneficial for the general population.

Systemic inflammation and endothelial dysfunction

Previous experimental studies have shown that diet-induced magnesium deficiency led to elevated serum concentrations of inflammatory cytokines in rodent models (Weglicki, Phillips et al. 1992; Weglicki, Dickens et al. 1996; Kurantsin-Mills, Cassidy et al. 1997; Kramer, Mak et al. 2003). Low-grade chronic inflammation, as reflected by elevated inflammatory markers, may be one of the common antecedents underlying the clustering of obesity, impaired glucose tolerance, dyslipidemia, and hypertension, known as the metabolic syndrome (Black, Kushner et al. 2004). Epidemiological data, though very limited, have provided some cross-sectional evidence linking magnesium intake to systemic inflammation as reflected by elevated concentrations of CRP. The inverse association between magnesium intake and CRP was first reported in a large population of 11,686 apparently healthy women in the WHS (Song, Ridker et al. 2005). In a large representative sample of US adults aged ≥20 years from the National Health and Nutrition Examination Survey 1999–2000, individuals who consumed less than the recommended daily allowance (RDA) of magnesium were 1.48–1.75 times more likely to have elevated CRP (≥3.0 mg/L) than those who consumed the RDA or more, after controlling for demographic and cardiovascular risk factors (King, Mainous et al. 2005). These findings are also supported by one cross-sectional study of 371 nondiabetic, normotensive obese Mexicans in whom serum magnesium concentrations were inversely associated with CRP concentrations (Guerrero-Romero and Rodriguez-Moran 2002) and a cross-sectional analysis of 657 women from the Nurses' Health Study (Song, Li et al. 2007). These consistent findings have led to the suggestion that the metabolic effects of magnesium intake might be, at least in part, due to its effects on systemic inflammation.

Although levels of CRP and endothelial adhesion molecules are not incorporated into the metabolic syndrome definitions being used, there is growing recognition that systemic inflammation and endothelial dysfunction may be two integral components of the metabolic syndrome. They are both common antecedents for the initiation of atherosclerosis and type 2 DM (Dandona, Aljada et al. 2005; Schram and Stehouwer 2005). Endothelial dysfunction has been closely related to insulin resistance (Pinkney, Stehouwer et al. 1997; Schram and Stehouwer 2005) and precedes the onset of early atherosclerotic cardiovascular disease and type 2 DM (Price and Loscalzo 1999). Magnesium may also have a direct effect on systemic inflammation and endothelial function. Some in vitro studies have shown that magnesium deficiency impaired the release of endothelial nitric oxide (Pearson, Evora et al. 1998) and enhanced free-radical-induced cytotoxicity in endothelial cells (Dickens, Weglicki et al. 1992), which in turn promoted endothelial dysfunction. One randomized, double-blind, placebo-controlled trial has shown that oral magnesium supplementation (30 mmol/d elemental magnesium) for six months resulted in a significant improvement in endothelium-dependent brachial artery flow-mediated vasodilation among 50 patients with coronary heart disease (Shechter, Sharir et al. 2000), indicating a direct effect of magnesium intake on endothelial function. Early endothelial dysfunction can readily be measured by circulating concentrations of endothelial soluble adhesion molecules. Because of limited data, it is unclear whether magnesium intake is inversely related to circulating concentrations of endothelial biomarkers. In addition, magnesium intake may have beneficial effects on other metabolic abnormalities that are not currently included in the conventionally diagnostic criteria for the metabolic syndrome such as its antioxidant, anti-arrhythmic, anticoagulant, or anti-platelet effects (Seelig and Heggtveit 1974; Altura and Altura 1995; Touyz 2004).

The metabolic syndrome

Metabolic syndrome comprises a constellation of metabolic abnormalities, including visceral obesity, glucose intolerance, hypertension, and dyslipidemia (Wilson and Grundy 2003a, 2003b). It is important to note that almost all epidemiologic studies of magnesium and the metabolic syndrome relied on the National Cholesterol Education Program (NCEP) Adult Treatment Program III (ATP III) diagnosis criteria (2001), although there are other commonly used diagnosis criteria, such as those of the World Health Organization (WHO) (Alberti and Zimmet 1998), the European Group on Insulin Resistance (EGIR) (Balkau and Charles 1999), the American Association of Clinical Endocrinologists (AACE) (Einhorn, Reaven et al. 2003), and the International Diabetes Federation (IDF) (Alberti, Zimmet et al. 2005). The evidence that magnesium favorably affects these metabolic abnormalities, though not entirely consistent, has led to a hypothesis that magnesium intake is related to a lower risk of metabolic syndrome. Regardless of diverse definitions used for the metabolic syndrome as an entity in different studies, this notion has been supported by epidemiologic evidence.

Two cross-sectional studies have related serum magnesium level to metabolic syndrome and/or its components. In a cross-sectional population-based study of 192 individuals with metabolic syndrome and 384 matched healthy control subjects, low serum magnesium levels were associated with elevated risk of metabolic syndrome defined by the presence of at least two of the features (hyperglycemia, high BP, elevated fasting triglycerides, low HDL-C, and obesity) (Guerrero-Romero and Rodriguez-Moran 2002). In another cross-sectional study, low levels of serum-ionized magnesium were associated with the metabolic syndrome, and serum magnesium level was inversely related to triglycerides and waist circumference. However, it remains controversial whether serum magnesium levels can reflect long-term magnesium intake or total magnesium status in the human body (Reinhart 1988). Serum magnesium did not appear to be correlated well with dietary magnesium intake and the intracellular magnesium pool; a biologically active portion of magnesium stores (Reinhart 1988; Liao, Folsom et al. 1998).

Magnesium intake has been observed to be associated with all the features of the metabolic syndrome. Song et al. first reported an inverse relation between dietary intake of magnesium and the prevalence of metabolic syndrome among 11,686 apparently healthy American women in the Women's Health Study (Song, Manson et al. 2004). Compared with those who are in the lowest quintile of magnesium intake, women in the highest quintile of intake had 27% lower risk of the metabolic syndrome according to the ATP-III criteria (OR: 0.73; 95% CI: 0.60–0.88; p for trend < 0.001). This inverse association also appeared to be more pronounced among women who were overweight and those who had ever smoked. The authors suggested that a possible beneficial effect of magnesium intake on diabetes and cardiovascular disease might be related to its roles in ameliorating systemic inflammation and/or the development of the metabolic syndrome. Using data from the NHANES III, Ford et al. provided consistent evidence from a cross-sectional analysis that magnesium intake is inversely associated with the prevalence of the metabolic syndrome in both men and women (Ford, Li et al. 2007). The multivariable OR of metabolic syndrome (according to the criteria of the ATP-III) for participants in the highest quintile of magnesium intake was 0.56 (95% CI: 0.34–0.92; p for trend = 0.029) compared with those who in the lowest quintile of intake. The results held after vitamin or mineral supplement users were excluded.

Recently, He et al. conducted a longitudinal study and prospectively examined the relations between magnesium intake and incident metabolic syndrome and its components (defined by the ATP-III definition) in young American adults (He, Liu et al. 2006). During the 15 years of follow-up, the investigators documented 608 incident cases of the metabolic syndrome among 4,637 Americans, aged 18 to 30 years, who were free from metabolic syndrome and diabetes at the baseline. After adjustment for potential confounders and baseline status of each component of the metabolic syndrome, magnesium intake was inversely associated with incidence of metabolic syndrome. The multivariable hazard ratio of metabolic syndrome for participants in the highest quartile was 0.69 (95% CI: 0.52–0.91; p for trend < 0.01) compared with those in the lowest quartile of magnesium intake. The inverse associations were not appreciably modified by gender and race (Caucasian and African American). Especially, significant inverse relations were also observed between magnesium intake and fasting glucose level, waist circumference, and HDL cholesterol.

Collectively, cross-sectional evidence has shown that magnesium intake correlates significantly with features of the metabolic syndrome (or insulin resistance syndrome), including adiposity, hyperinsulinemia, insulin resistance, hypertriglyceridemia, and low HDL cholesterol and hypertension (Fung, Manson et al. 2003; Song, Ridker et al. 2005). Magnesium intake may also have beneficial effects on other metabolic abnormalities that are not currently included in the conventionally diagnosis criteria for the metabolic syndrome such as systemic inflammation and endothelial dysfunction. The metabolic syndrome is now reaching epidemic proportions worldwide and may reflect a common underlying pathophysiology related to chronic diseases including type 2 DM (Colditz, Manson et al. 1992; Salmeron, Ascherio et al. 1997; Song, Manson et al. 2004), cardiovascular disease (Abbott, Ando et al. 2003; Al-Delaimy, Rimm et al. 2004; Song, Manson et al. 2005), hypertension (Ascherio, Rimm et al. 1992; Song, Sesso et al. 2006), and colorectal cancer (Larsson, Bergkvist et al. 2005; Folsom and Hong 2006).

Magnesium intake and type 2 DM

A large body of data from clinical case studies and cross-sectional studies provided further evidence for the correlation between blood magnesium levels and type 2 DM (Mather, Nisbet et al. 1979; Levin, Mather et al. 1981; McNair, Christensen et al. 1982; Yajnik, Smith et al. 1984; Paolisso, Scheen et al. 1990; Resnick, Altura et al. 1993; Alzaid, Dinneen et al. 1995; Ma, Folsom et al. 1995; Paolisso and Ravusin 1995). Hypomagnesemia is common among patients with diabetes, especially those with poor metabolic control (Mather, Nisbet et al. 1979; Sjogren, Floren et al. 1988; Resnick,

Altura et al. 1993). Polyuria caused by hyperglycemia, coupled with hyper-insulinemia, tended to increase renal excretion of magnesium or decrease renal re-absorption of magnesium, thereby resulting in hypomagnese-mia in type 2 DM (McNair, Christensen et al. 1982; Djurhuus, Skott et al. 1995). Inadequate intake of dietary magnesium in diabetic patients may also cause hypomagnesemia (Schmidt, Arfken et al. 1994). However, these results are inconclusive in testing the hypothesis regarding the role of magnesium due to confounding by other aspects of diet, physical activity, smoking, obesity, socioeconomic status, and drug therapies such as hypo-glycemic medication, diuretics, and insulin. Thus, whether low plasma magnesium is a cause or consequence of suboptimal glycemic control remains inconclusive.

Results from prospective studies of magnesium intake and risk of type 2 DM have been generally consistent. Previous reports from the Nurses' Health Study (Colditz, Manson et al. 1992; Salmeron, Manson et al. 1997), the Iowa Women's Health Study (Meyer, Kushi et al. 2000), the Health Professionals Follow-up Study (Salmeron, Ascherio et al. 1997), the European Prospective Investigation Into Cancer and Nutrition (EPIC)-Postdam Study (Schulze, Schulz et al. 2007), and the Black Women's Health Study (van Dam, Hu et al. 2006) all indicated an inverse association between magnesium intake and risk of incident type 2 DM, although such an association was not found in the ARIC study with a relatively small number of incident cases (Kao, Folsom et al. 1999). However, the prospec-tive ARIC study showed an inverse association between serum concentra-tions of magnesium at baseline and subsequent risk of type 2 DM (Kao, Folsom et al. 1999). Since there is a lack of correlation between serum lev-els and dietary magnesium intake (r = 0.06) (Elin 1987; Djurhuus, Gram et al. 1995; Kao, Folsom et al. 1999), such an association may not reflect the impact of long-term magnesium intake.

When the data from these prospective cohorts were pooled in a meta-analysis, the summary estimate of relative risk (RR) for type 2 DM was 0.76 comparing the highest category of dietary magnesium intake with the lowest category of intake (95% CI: 0.69–0.85; $P = 0.04$ for between-study heterogeneity). Our results were consistent with two recent meta-analyses that were independently conducted but did not include all the prospective studies available. In one meta-analysis of eight independent cohorts with 286,668 participants and 10912 diabetes cases, the overall RR for a 100 mg/day increase in magnesium intake was 0.85 (95% CI, 0.79–0.92; $P = 0.002$ for between-study heterogeneity). Results were similar for dietary mag-nesium (RR, 0.86; 95% CI, 0.77–0.95) and total magnesium (RR, 0.83; 95% CI, 0.77–0.89) (Larsson and Wolk 2007). In another separate meta-analysis of eight cohorts involving 271,869 participants and 9,792 cases, the RR for the highest category compared with the lowest category was 0.77 (95%CI, 0.72–0.84; $P = 0.04$ for between-study heterogeneity) for total magnesium intake (Schulze, Schulz et al. 2007). Although cereal fiber is highly cor-related with magnesium intake and may explain in part the observed beneficial effect of magnesium intake, cereal fiber has been associated with a lower diabetes risk independent of magnesium in several previ-ous cohort studies and meta-analyses (He, Liu et al. 2006; van Dam, Hu et al. 2006; Schulze, Schulz et al. 2007). Thus, the evidence from prospective cohort studies is strongly supportive of the role of magnesium intake in the development of type 2 DM.

In an earlier report from the Nurses' Health Study, women in the highest quintile compared with the lowest quintile of magnesium intake had a RR of 0.68 (95% confidence interval [CI], 0.45–1.01; P for trend = 0.02) for women with a BMI less than 29 and 0.73 (95% CI, 0.53–1.02; P for trend = 0.008) for women with a BMI of 29 or higher (Colditz, Manson et al. 1992). In another large cohort of 39,345 middle-aged and older US women participating in the Women's Health Study with an average of 6-year fol-low-up, this inverse association remained significant albeit only among women with a BMI of 25 or more (RR, 0.78; 95% CI, 0.62–0.99; P for trend = 0.02) (Song, Manson et al. 2004). Because the extent to which magnesium intake influences insulin sensitivity may differ among women with dif-ferent body fat, we speculated that the potential beneficial effects of high intake of magnesium may be greater among overweight persons who are prone to insulin resistance. It remains to be confirmed in future studies whether magnesium intake has differential beneficial effects in individu-als with different levels of metabolic status.

There are as yet no clinical trials examining the efficacy of magne-sium supplementation or consumption of major magnesium-rich foods on the primary prevention of type 2 DM. In the 1980s, several nonrandom-ized and uncontrolled trials for secondary prevention in diabetic patients showed that oral magnesium supplementation may improve glucose tol-erance and reduce insulin requirement among patients with type 2 DM (Karppanen, Tanskanen et al. 1984; Sjogren, Floren et al. 1988; Gullestad, Jacobsen et al. 1994; Yokota, Kato et al. 2004). Nine randomized controlled trials of oral magnesium supplementation have assessed diabetes-related phenotypes (e.g., glycemic control, or insulin sensitivity) among patients with type 2 DM (Paolisso, Sgambato et al. 1989; Gullestad, Jacobsen et al. 1994; Paolisso, Scheen et al. 1994; Purvis, Cummings et al. 1994; Eibl, Kopp et al. 1995; Eriksson and Kohvakka 1995; de Lourdes Lima, Cruz et al. 1998; de Valk, Verkaaik et al. 1998; Rodriguez-Moran and Guerrero-Romero 2003). A total of 370 patients with type 2 DM were enrolled in these 9 trials evaluating oral magnesium supplementation (median dose: 15 mmol/day [360 mg/day]) from 4 to 16 weeks (median: 12 weeks) to improve diabetes control. Of them, four randomized double-blind trials showed beneficial effects by oral magnesium supplementation on glycemic control among patients with type 2 diabetes (Paolisso, Sgambato et al. 1989; Paolisso,

Scheen et al. 1994; de Lourdes Lima, Cruz et al. 1998; Rodriguez-Moran and Guerrero-Romero 2003). By contrast, five randomized double-blind placebo-controlled trials showed no beneficial effects of oral magnesium supplementation on glycemic control among patients with type 2 DM (Gullestad, Jacobsen et al. 1994; Purvis, Cummings et al. 1994; Eibl, Kopp et al. 1995; Eriksson and Kohvakka 1995; de Valk, Verkaaik et al. 1998). Because almost all trials included small numbers of participants and were of relatively short duration, these randomized controlled trials have been underpowered to reliably assess the efficacy of oral magnesium supplementation. In addition, differences in study population, duration of diabetes, glycemic treatment, and intervention periods, coupled with different magnesium doses and formulations used, have led to difficulties in interpreting the potential benefits of oral magnesium supplementation for patients with type 2 DM. Oral magnesium supplementation as adjunct therapy may be effective in improving glycemic control among type 2 DM patients. Side effects were relatively infrequent among diabetic patients in the magnesium treatment group. No severe adverse effects, including cardiovascular events or deaths, were reported. The most common side effects were gastrointestinal symptoms, including diarrhea and abdominal pain (Paolisso, Sgambato et al. 1989; Gullestad, Jacobsen et al. 1994; Paolisso, Scheen et al. 1994; Purvis, Cummings et al. 1994; Eibl, Kopp et al. 1995; Eriksson and Kohvakka 1995; de Lourdes Lima, Cruz et al. 1998; de Valk, Verkaaik et al. 1998; Rodriguez-Moran and Guerrero-Romero 2003). However, the long-term benefits and safety of magnesium treatment on glycemic control remain to be determined in future large-scale, well-designed randomized controlled trials with long follow-up periods.

Multivitamin use and type 2 DM

Multivitamin supplements contain large amounts of many vitamins and minerals that approximate or exceed the recommended micronutrient intakes. With the relative safety and inexpensiveness, multivitamin supplements are the most commonly used dietary supplements in the United States and are advocated as an attractive option for preventing chronic diseases, such as cancer, cardiovascular disease, and type 2 DM (2006; Rock 2007). Approximately 50% of US adults routinely take multivitamin supplements and spend about $23 billion on these supplements each year in the United States (2006). Data from the National Health and Nutrition Examination Survey (NHANES) have shown a trend of increasing use of multivitamin supplements in the general population of the United States. Multivitamin supplement use may contribute a considerable proportion of nutrient intakes in most dietary supplement users and may contribute to the risk of excessive intakes of micronutrients in some subgroups (Rock 2007). Despite the widespread use of multivitamins in the US population, few epidemiologic studies have been available evaluating the overall benefit and risks of multivitamins for chronic disease prevention.

With their popularity, multivitamin supplement use contributes to a considerable proportion of micronutrient intakes among users and sometimes excessive intakes of certain micronutrients in some subgroups of the population (Rock 2007). There is a long-standing interest in the diabetes research community regarding the potential yet unproven benefits or risks of multivitamin use on the development and progression of type 2 diabetes. However, most epidemiologic studies on vitamins and diabetes risk to date have focused on individual vitamins. Evidence from basic research and observational studies has suggested that adequate intake of antioxidant vitamin or minerals may protect against the development of type 2 diabetes via reduction of oxidative stress and its associated metabolic abnormalities including systemic inflammation, endothelial dysfunction, hypertension, and dyslipidemia (Paolisso, Balbi et al. 1995; Mullan, Young et al. 2002; Regensteiner, Popylisen et al. 2003). These metabolic abnormalities act individually or synergistically to impair pancreatic β-cell insulin secretion and interfere with glucose disposal in peripheral tissues (Ceriello and Motz 2004), thereby accelerating the development and progression of both atherosclerosis and type 2 diabetes. A recent study also showed that multivitamin use is associated with longer telomere length, which is a reliable marker of biological aging as a result of multiple metabolic disorders, especially oxidative stress and chronic inflammation (Xu, Parks et al. 2009).

Despite a lack of consistent evidence on the effects of individual nutrient supplements on preventing diabetes, few prospective studies have specifically evaluated the potential benefits and risks of long-term multivitamin use in preventing type 2 DM. Recent data from the National Institute of Health-AARP Diet and Health (NIH-AARP DH) cohort found no significant association between multivitamin use and diabetes risk (Song, Xu et al. 2011). Use of vitamin E or other individual vitamin and mineral supplements (including iron, zinc, selenium, folic acid, vitamin A, and β-carotene) were not associated with diabetes risk, whereas the findings of lower diabetes risk among frequent users of vitamin C or calcium supplements need to be further evaluated. Due to the exploratory and observational nature of this study, the potential benefit of multivitamin use on diabetes prevention should be further evaluated in future longitudinal studies or randomized trials.

Possible synergistic effects of micronutrients

Antioxidants are members of a rather large and actively cooperating family of phytochemical substances. Synergistic interactions between antioxidants have been described in many experimental studies and may, in

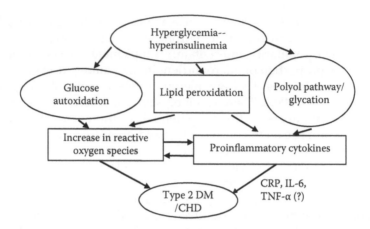

Figure 5.4 Schematic representation for hyperglycemia—oxidative/inflammatory pathways.

part, involve the regeneration of antioxidants. For example, a certain level of vitamin E may be sufficient when the levels of all the other antioxidants are sufficient, but the protective effect of that level of vitamin E may become inadequate when levels of other antioxidants fall (Gey 1994). It is important, therefore, to examine the interaction between vitamin E and vitamin C on reducing the risk of type 2 DM.

As shown in Figure 5.4, reactive oxygen species are produced as part of the inflammatory process. Both endogenous and exogenous sources of antioxidants serve to counteract the reactive oxygen species, thus limiting or preventing cellular or subcellular damage by free radicals. Unless the pools of antioxidants are replenished (through increased intake or endogenous production), the increase in reactive oxygen species from inflammation may deplete these pools resulting in lower concentrations of antioxidants, which in turn aggravates the oxidation/inflammatory processes. Thus, it would be of interest to examine whether trials of antioxidant supplementation would be more effective among those with elevated C-reactive protein concentration. On the other hand, higher antioxidant concentrations could reduce inflammation because sufficient supplies of antioxidants could conceivably mitigate the inflammatory process at critical points. Reactive oxygen species and lipid peroxidation can promote the production of proinflammatory cytokines. By neutralizing free radicals, increased concentrations of antioxidants could directly reduce one stimulus for increases in proinflammatory cytokines and indirectly reduce a second stimulus by reducing lipid peroxidation. For example, oxidized LDL cholesterol is a stimulus of inflammation (Massy 2000; Massy, Kim et al. 2000). If antioxidants could prevent or reduce the oxidation of LDL cholesterol, some of the inflammatory stimulus could be reduced. This would suggest that an adequate supply of antioxidants may be especially critical in preventing the early development of type 2 DM.

Using a large representative sample of US adults in NHANES III, investigators have recently found that C-reactive protein concentration is inversely associated with concentrations of vitamin C, vitamin E, folate, carotenoids, and selenium, irrespective of age, sex, race, or ethnicity (Kritchevsky, Bush et al. 2000; Ford, Liu et al. 2001). Compared to participants in the lowest quartile of plasma vitamin C, those who were in the highest quartile had a 44% (95% CI, 31%-54%, *P* for trend, <0.01) lower risk of elevated hs-CRP (defined as >85th percentile of the general population). Other studies have examined some of these relationships in samples of individuals with various conditions. In a study of 85 nuns aged 77–99 years, hs-CRP concentrations were inversely related to plasma concentrations of α-carotene, ß-carotene, lycopene, and total carotenoids (Boosalis, Snowdon et al. 1996). Among 57 individuals with type 2 DM, vitamin E supplementation of 800 IU/day resulted in decreases of hs-CRP concentrations (Upritchard, Sutherland et al. 2000). Inverse relationships between hs-CRP concentrations and retinol, vitamin C, tocopherol, and lutein have also been noted among individuals with lung cancer (Talwar, Ha et al. 1997), acute pancreatitis (Curran, Sattar et al. 2000), and those undergoing orthopedic surgery (Louw, Werbeck et al. 1992). Furthermore, vitamins A, C, and E decrease transiently during the course of an acute myocardial infarction (Labadarios, Brink et al. 1987). Patients with gastrointestinal cancer and an elevated hs-CRP concentration had lower concentrations of vitamins and minerals than similar patients with normal hs-CRP concentrations (McMillan, Sattar et al. 2000). Taken together, these findings suggest that it may be possible to temper the underlying inflammatory process of atherosclerosis or perhaps limit the secondary damage from increased oxidative stress caused by inflammatory processes by dietary modification (Figure 5.3). Because many antioxidants are found in fruits, vegetables, and whole grains, these data also provide a mechanism for the action of some of the antioxidant nutrients contained in these foods in preventing type 2 DM or CHD. Additional studies are needed to examine the relationships between inflammatory markers and antioxidant concentrations and to determine causality. For example, supplementation studies in persons with elevated hs-CRP may reveal whether antioxidants may have an effect on the inflammatory process and which ones are more likely to be effective. However, no randomized trial data are available to evaluate the possibility of a synergistic relationship between aspirin and vitamin E in the prevention of type 2 DM. Although observational studies have indicated that a diet rich in whole grains, fruits, and vegetables is associated with lower oxidative stress and reduced risk of both type 2 DM and CHD, only population-based randomized intervention trials will ultimately determine the efficacy of an antioxidant cocktail in the primary prevention of these degenerative diseases of aging.

Summary

Given the increasing public health impact of type 2 DM in the United States and around the world, the identification of effective and safe preventive measures that offer even modest reductions in incidence could have a significant public health impact. Antioxidant vitamins, anti-inflammatory drugs, and homocysteine-lowering agents represent three such promising interventions (American Diabetes Association 1998). However, considerable uncertainty exists regarding the efficacy of these intervention agents, and current epidemiologic and clinical data cannot provide definitive answers regarding their use in the primary prevention of type 2 DM. A major problem is the lack of long-term, large-scale randomized clinical trials. When examining exposures such as aspirin use or vitamin supplementation using an observational design, selection and confounding biases can easily affect any material findings and produce spurious interpretation. Thus, observational studies are not likely to provide any definitive answer regarding the balance of benefits or risks associated with the use of these interventions. Because of the null findings regarding the effects of vitamin E in the secondary prevention of CVD from both the HOPE and GISSI trials, it seems unlikely that a new trial would be initiated to answer the scientific questions regarding the efficacy of antioxidant vitamins in the primary prevention of type 2 DM. The existence of ongoing and complementary randomized trials already testing these preventive strategies for CVD and cancer provides a unique opportunity to provide timely answers regarding these possible preventive agents for type 2 DM at a fraction of the cost of initiating new trials. Findings from these three trials, no matter whether they are positive or negative, will provide a rational basis for informed clinical decision making for individuals as well as policy recommendations for the health of the general public.

References

Abbasi, F., F. Facchini et al. (1999). "Plasma homocysteine concentrations in healthy volunteers are not related to differences in insulin-mediated glucose disposal." *Atherosclerosis* 146(1): 175–178.
Abbott, R. D., F. Ando et al. (2003). "Dietary magnesium intake and the future risk of coronary heart disease (the Honolulu Heart Program)." *Am J Cardiol* 92(6): 665–669.
Al-Delaimy, W. K., E. B. Rimm et al. (2004). "Magnesium intake and risk of coronary heart disease among men." *J Am Coll Nutr* 23(1): 63–70.

Alberti, K. G., P. Zimmet et al. (2005). "The metabolic syndrome—a new world-wide definition." *Lancet* **366**(9491): 1059–1062.

Alberti, K. G. and P. Z. Zimmet (1998). "Definition, diagnosis and classification of diabetes mellitus and its complications. Part 1: Diagnosis and classification of diabetes mellitus provisional report of a WHO consultation." *Diabet Med* **15**(7): 539–553.

Altura, B. M. and B. T. Altura (1995). "Magnesium and cardiovascular biology: An important link between cardiovascular risk factors and atherogenesis." *Cell Mol Biol Res* **41**(5): 347–359.

Altura, B. T., M. Brust et al. (1990). "Magnesium dietary intake modulates blood lipid levels and atherogenesis." *Proc Natl Acad Sci U S A* **87**(5): 1840–1844.

Alzaid, A. A., S. F. Dinneen et al. (1995). "Effects of insulin on plasma magnesium in noninsulin-dependent diabetes mellitus: Evidence for insulin resistance." *J Clin Endocrinol Metab.* **80**: 1376–1381.

American Diabetes Association (1997). "Aspirin therapy in diabetes." *Diabetes care* **20**: 1772–1773.

American Diabetes Association (1998). "Nutritional recommendations and principles for individuals with diabetes mellitus." *Diabetes Care* **21**: 532–535.

Ames, B., M. Shigenaga et al. (1993). "Oxidants, antioxidants, and the degenerative diseases of aging." *Proc Natl Acad Sci USA* **90**: 7915–7922.

Ammon, H. P., S. Klumpp et al. (1989). "A possible role of plasma glutathione in glucose-mediated insulin secretion: In vitro and in vivo studies in rats." *Diabetologia* **32**(11): 797–800.

Araki, A., Y. Sako et al. (1993). "Plasma homocysteine concentrations in Japanese patients with non-insulin-dependent diabetes mellitus: Effect of parenteral methylcobalamin treatment." *Atherosclerosis* **103**(2): 149–157.

Ascherio, A., C. Hennekens et al. (1996). "Prospective study of nutritional factors, blood pressure, and hypertension among US women." *Hypertension* **27**(5): 1065–1072.

Ascherio, A., E. B. Rimm et al. (1992). "A prospective study of nutritional factors and hypertension among US men." *Circulation* **86**(5): 1475–1484.

Baigent, C. and R. Clarke (2007). "B vitamins for the prevention of vascular disease: Insufficient evidence to justify treatment." *JAMA* **298**(10): 1212–1214.

Balkau, B. and M. A. Charles (1999). "Comment on the provisional report from the WHO consultation. European Group for the Study of Insulin Resistance (EGIR)." *Diabet Med* **16**(5): 442–443.

Barbagallo, M., L. J. Dominguez et al. (2003). "Role of magnesium in insulin action, diabetes and cardio-metabolic syndrome X." *Mol Aspects Med* **24**: 39–52.

Baynes, J. W. and S. R. Thorpe (1999). "Role of oxidative stress in diabetic complications: A new perspective on an old paradigm." *Diabetes* **48**(1): 1–9.

Bazzano, L. A., K. Reynolds et al. (2006). "Effect of folic acid supplementation on risk of cardiovascular diseases: A meta-analysis of randomized controlled trials." *JAMA* **296**(22): 2720–2726.

Beales, P. E., A. J. Williams et al. (1994). "Vitamin E delays diabetes onset in the non-obese diabetic mouse." *Horm Metab Res* **26**(10): 450–452.

Beaulieu, C., R. Kostckian et al. (1993). "Calcium is essential in normalizing intolerance to glucose that accompanies vitamin D depletion in vivo." *Diabetes* **42**(1): 35–43.

Billaudel, B., A. Faure et al. (1989). "Direct in vitro effect of 1,25-dihydroxyvitamin D3 on islets insulin secretion in vitamin deficient rats: Influence of vitamin D3 pretreatment." *Diabete Metab* **15**(2): 85–87.

Bischoff-Ferrari, H. A., E. Giovannucci et al. (2006). "Estimation of optimal serum concentrations of 25-hydroxyvitamin D for multiple health outcomes." *Am J Clin Nutr* **84**(1): 18–28.

Black, S., I. Kushner et al. (2004). "C-reactive protein." *J Biol Chem* **279**(47): 48487–48490.

Bloomgarden, Z. (1997). "Antioxidants and diabetes." *Diabetes Care* **20**: 670–673.

Boosalis, M. G., D. A. Snowdon et al. (1996). "Acute phase response and plasma carotenoid concentrations in older women: Findings from the nun study." *Nutrition* **12**(7–8): 475–478.

Boucher, B. J. (1998). "Inadequate vitamin D status: Does it contribute to the disorders comprising syndrome 'X'?" *Br J Nutr* **79**(4): 315–327.

Boucher, B. J., N. Mannan et al. (1995). "Glucose intolerance and impairment of insulin secretion in relation to vitamin D deficiency in east London Asians." *Diabetologia* **38**(10): 1239–1245.

Boushey, C. J., S. A. A. Beresford et al. (1995). "A quantitative assessment of plasma homocysteine as a risk factor for vascular disease: Probable benefits of increasing folic acid intakes." *J Am Med Assoc* **274**: 1049–1057.

Brattstrom, L. (1996). "Vitamins as homocysteine lowering agents." *J Nutr* **126**: 1276S–1280S.

Brattstrom, L., B. Israelsson et al. (1990). "Impaired homocysteine metabolism in early-onset cerebral and peripheral occlusive arterial disease: Effects of pyridoxine and folic acid treatment." *Atherosclerosis* **81**: 51–60.

Brattstrom, L. E., B. Israelsson et al. (1988). "Folic acid: An innocuous means to reduce plasma homocyst(e)ine." *Scand J Clin Lab Invest* **48**: 215–221.

Bunn, H. F. (1981). "Evaluation of glycosylated hemoglobin diabetic patients." *Diabetes* **30**: 613–617.

Caballero, A. E. (2003). "Endothelial dysfunction in obesity and insulin resistance: A road to diabetes and heart disease." *Obes Res* **11**(11): 1278–1289.

Caballero, B. (1993). "Vitamin E improves the action of insulin." *Nutr Rev* **51**: 339–340.

Cade, C. and A. W. Norman (1986). "Vitamin D3 improves impaired glucose tolerance and insulin secretion in the vitamin D-deficient rat in vivo." *Endocrinology* **119**(1): 84–90.

Carantoni, M., F. Abbasi et al. (1998). "Relationship between insulin resistance and partially oxidized LDL particles in healthy, nondiabetic volunteers." *Arterioscler Thromb Vasc Biol* **18**(5): 762–767.

Ceriello, A., D. Giugliano et al. (1991). "Vitamin E reduction of protein glycosylation in diabetes. New prospect for prevention of diabetic complications?" *Diabetes Care* **14**(1): 68–72.

Ceriello, A. and E. Motz (2004). "Is oxidative stress the pathogenic mechanism underlying insulin resistance, diabetes, and cardiovascular disease? The common soil hypothesis revisited." *Arterioscler Thromb Vasc Biol* **24**(5): 816–823.

Chakraborti, S., T. Chakraborti et al. (2002). "Protective role of magnesium in cardiovascular diseases: A review." *Mol Cell Biochem* **238**(1–2): 163–179.

Chisolm, G. M., K. C. Irwin et al. (1992). "Lipoprotein oxidation and lipoprotein-induced cell injury in diabetes." *Diabetes* **41** Suppl 2: 61–66.

Chiu, K. C., A. Chu et al. (2004). "Hypovitaminosis D is associated with insulin resistance and beta cell dysfunction." *Am J Clin Nutr* **79**(5): 820–825.

Cho, N. H., S. Lim et al. (2005). "Elevated homocysteine as a risk factor for the development of diabetes in women with a previous history of gestational diabetes mellitus: A 4-year prospective study." *Diabetes Care* **28**(11): 2750–2755.

Choi, H. K., W. C. Willett et al. (2005). "Dairy consumption and risk of type 2 diabetes mellitus in men: A prospective study." *Arch Intern Med* **165**(9): 997–1003.

Cleveland, L. E., J. D. Goldman et al. (1994). *Data tables: Results from USDA's 1994 continuing survey of food intakes by individuals and 1994 diet and health knowledge survey.* Beltsville, MD., Agricultural Research Service, U.S. Department of Agriculture.

Clopath, P., V. Smith et al. (1976). "Growth promotion by homocysteic acid." *Science* **192**: 372–374.

Colditz, G. A., J. E. Manson et al. (1992). "Diet and risk of clinical diabetes in women." *Am J Clin Nutr* **55**(5): 1018–1023.

Colewell, J. (1997). "Aspirin therapy in diabetes." *Diabetes Care* **20**: 1767–1771.

Cooke, J. P. and P. S. Tsao (1993). "Cytoprotective effects of nitric oxide." *Circulation* **88**(5 Pt 1): 2451–2454.

Curran, F. J., N. Sattar et al. (2000). "Relationship of carotenoid and vitamins A and E with the acute inflammatory response in acute pancreatitis." *Br J Surg* **87**(3): 301–305.

Dandona, P., A. Aljada et al. (2005). "Metabolic syndrome: a comprehensive perspective based on interactions between obesity, diabetes, and inflammation." *Circulation* **111**(11): 1448–1454.

Dandona, P., K. Thusu et al. (1996). "Oxidative damage to DNA in diabetes mellitus." *Lancet* **347**(8999): 444–445.

Das, S., T. Reynolds et al. (1999). "Plasma homocysteine concentrations in type II diabetic patients in India: Relationship to body weight." *J Diabetes Complications* **13**(4): 200–203.

Davis, C. D. and J. T. Dwyer (2007). "The 'sunshine vitamin': Benefits beyond bone?" *J Natl Cancer Inst* **99**(21): 1563–1565.

Davis, R. E., J. S. Calder et al. (1976). "Serum pyridoxal and folate concentrations in diabetics." *Pathology* **8**(2): 151–156.

Dawson-Hughes, B., R. P. Heaney et al. (2005). "Estimates of optimal vitamin D status." *Osteoporos Int* **16**(7): 713–716.

Dawson, E. B., M. J. Frey et al. (1978). "Relationship of metal metabolism to vascular disease mortality rates in Texas." *Am J Clin Nutr* **31**(7): 1188–1197.

de Boer, I. H., L. F. Tinker et al. (2008). "Calcium plus vitamin D supplementation and the risk of incident diabetes in the Women's Health Initiative." *Diabetes Care* **31**(4): 701–707.

de Lourdes Lima, M., T. Cruz et al. (1998). "The effect of magnesium supplementation in increasing doses on the control of type 2 diabetes." *Diabetes Care* **21**: 682–686.

de Valk, H. W., R. Verkaaik et al. (1998). "Oral magnesium supplementation in insulin requiring type 2 diabetic patients." *Diabetes Med* **15**: 503–507.

DerSimonian, R. and N. M. Laird (1986). "Meta-analysis in clinical trials." *Control Clin Trials* **7**: 177–188.

Dickens, B. F., W. B. Weglicki et al. (1992). "Magnesium deficiency in vitro enhances free radical-induced intracellular oxidation and cytotoxicity in endothelial cells." *FEBS Lett* **311**(3): 187–191.

Djurhuus, M. S., J. Gram et al. (1995). "Biological variation of serum and urinary magnesium in apparently healthy males." *Scand J Clin Lab Invest* **55**(6): 549–558.

Djurhuus, M. S., P. Skott et al. (1995). "Insulin increases renal magnesium excretion: A possible cause of magnesium depletion in hyperinsulinaemic states." *Diabet Med* **12**(8): 664–669.

Eibl, N. L., H. P. Kopp et al. (1995). "Hypomagnesemia in type II diabetes: Effect of a 3-month replacement therapy." *Diabetes Care* **18**: 188–192.

Einhorn, D., G. M. Reaven et al. (2003). "American College of Endocrinology position statement on the insulin resistance syndrome." *Endocr Pract* **9**(3): 237–252.

Elin, R. J. (1987). "Assessment of magnesium status." *Clin Chem* **33**(11): 1965–1970.

Elwood, P. C., J. E. Pickering et al. (2007). "Milk and dairy consumption, diabetes and the metabolic syndrome: The Caerphilly prospective study." *J Epidemiol Community Health* **61**(8): 695–698.

Eriksson, J. and A. Kohvakka (1995). "Magnesium and ascorbic acid supplementation in diabetes mellitus." *Ann Nutr Metab* **39**(4): 217–223.

Evans, J. L., I. D. Goldfine et al. (2003). "Are oxidative stress-activated signaling pathways mediators of insulin resistance and beta-cell dysfunction?" *Diabetes* **52**(1): 1–8.

Facchini, F. S., N. W. Hua et al. (2000). "Hyperinsulinemia: The missing link among oxidative.

Facchini, F. S., M. H. Humphreys et al. (2000). "Relation between insulin resistance and plasma concentrations of lipid hydroperoxides, carotenoids, and tocopherols." *Am J Clin Nutr* **72**(3): 776–779.

Fang, Y., J. B. van Meurs et al. (2005). "Promoter and 3'-untranslated-region haplotypes in the vitamin d receptor gene predispose to osteoporotic fracture: The rotterdam study." *Am J Hum Genet* **77**(5): 807–823.

Feskens, E. J., S. M. Virtanen et al. (1995). "Dietary factors determining diabetes and impaired glucose tolerance. A 20-year follow-up of the Finnish and Dutch cohorts of the Seven Countries Study." *Diabetes Care* **18**(8): 1104–1112.

Fliser, D., A. Stefanski et al. (1997). "No effect of calcitriol on insulin-mediated glucose uptake in healthy subjects." *Eur J Clin Invest* **27**(7): 629–633.

Folsom, A. R. and C. P. Hong (2006). "Magnesium intake and reduced risk of colon cancer in a prospective study of women." *Am J Epidemiol* **163**(3): 232–235.

Fonseca, V. A., L. M. Fink et al. (2003). "Insulin sensitivity and plasma homocysteine concentrations in non-diabetic obese and normal weight subjects." *Atherosclerosis* **167**(1): 105–109.

Fonseca, V. A., S. Mudaliar et al. (1998). "Plasma homocysteine concentrations are regulated by acute hyperinsulinemia in nondiabetic but not type 2 diabetic subjects." *Metabolism* **47**(6): 686–689.

Fonseca, V. A., A. Stone et al. (1997). "Oxidative stress in diabetic macrovascular disease: Does homocysteine play a role?" *South Med J* **90**(9): 903–906.

Ford, E., S. Liu et al. (2001). "C-reactive protein concentration and concentrations of blood vitamins, carotenoids, and selenium among United States adults." *Am J Clin Nutr* Submitted.

Ford, E. S. (2001). "Vitamin supplement use and diabetes mellitus incidence among adults in the United States." *Am J Epidemiol* **153**(9): 892–897.

Ford, E. S., U. A. Ajani et al. (2005). "Concentrations of serum vitamin D and the metabolic syndrome among U.S. adults." *Diabetes Care* **28**(5): 1228–1230.

Ford, E. S., C. Li et al. (2007). "Intake of dietary magnesium and the prevalence of the metabolic syndrome among U.S. adults." *Obesity (Silver Spring)* **15**(5): 1139–1146.

Ford, E. S. and A. H. Mokdad (2003). "Dietary magnesium intake in a national sample of US adults." *J Nutr* **133**(9): 2879–2882.

Ford, E. S., J. C. Will et al. (1999). "Diabetes mellitus and serum carotenoids: Findings from the Third National Health and Nutrition Examination Survey." *Am J Epidemiol* **149**(2): 168–176.

Forouhi, N. G., J. Luan et al. (2008). "Baseline serum 25-hydroxy vitamin D is predictive of future glycemic status and insulin resistance: The Medical Research Council Ely Prospective Study 1990–2000." *Diabetes* **57**(10): 2619–2625.

Frei, B. (1994a). "Reactive oxygen species and antioxidant vitamins: Mechanisms of action." *Am J Med* **97**(Suppl.): 5S–13S.

Frei, B., Ed. (1994b). *Natural Antioxidants in Human Health and Disease.* New York, Academic Press.

Fung, T. T., J. E. Manson et al. (2003). "The association between magnesium intake and fasting insulin concentration in healthy middle-aged women." *J Am Coll Nutr* **22**(6): 533–538.

Gedik, O. and S. Akalin (1986). "Effects of vitamin D deficiency and repletion on insulin and glucagon secretion in man." *Diabetologia* **29**(3): 142–145.

Gey, K. F. (1994). "Optimum plasma levels of antioxidant micronutrients. Ten years of antioxidant hypothesis on arteriosclerosis." *Bibliotheca Nutritio et Dieta* **51**: 84–99.

Giovannucci, E. (2005). "The epidemiology of vitamin D and cancer incidence and mortality: A review (United States)." *Cancer Causes Control* **16**(2): 83–95.

Giovannucci, E. (2009). "Expanding roles of vitamin D." *J Clin Endocrinol Metab* **94**(2): 418–420.

Giugliano, D., A. Ceriello et al. (1996). "Oxidative stress and diabetic vascular complications." *Diabetes Care* **19**(3): 257–267.

Giugliano, D., G. Paolisso et al. (1996). "Oxidative stress and diabetic vascular complications." *Diabetes Care* **19**: 257–267.

Gloth, F. M., C. M. Gundberg et al. (1995). "Vitamin D deficiency in homebound elderly persons." *JAMA* **274**(21): 1683–1686.

Godsland, I. F., J. R. Rosankiewicz et al. (2001). "Plasma total homocysteine concentrations are unrelated to insulin sensitivity and components of the metabolic syndrome in healthy men." *J Clin Endocrinol Metab* **86**(2): 719–723.

Golay, A. and J. Felber (1994). "Evolution from obesity to diabetes." *Diabetes Metab* **20**: 3–14.

Groff, J. L. and S. S. Gropper (2000). Macrominerals. In: *Advanced Nutrition and Human Metabolism.*, California, Wadsworth, 371–400.

Guerrero-Romero, F. and M. Rodriguez-Moran (2002a). "Low serum magnesium levels and metabolic syndrome." *Acta Diabetol* **39**(4): 209–213.

Guerrero-Romero, F. and M. Rodriguez-Moran (2002b). "Relationship between serum magnesium levels and C-reactive protein concentration, in non-diabetic, non-hypertensive obese subjects." *Int J Obes Relat Metab Disord* **26**(4): 469–474.

Guerrero-Romero, F., H. E. Tamez-Perez et al. (2004). "Oral magnesium supplementation improves insulin sensitivity in non-diabetic subjects with insulin resistance. A double-blind placebo-controlled randomized trial." *Diabetes Metab* 30(3): 253–258.

Gullestad, L., T. Jacobsen et al. (1994). "Effect of magnesium treatment on glycemic control and metabolic parameters in NIDDM patients." *Diabetes Care* 17(5): 460–461.

Haffner, S., M. Stern et al. (1990). "Incidence of type II diabetes in Mexican Americans predicted by fasting insulin and glucose levels, obesity, and body-fat distribution." *Diabetes* 39: 283–288.

Hajer, G. R., Y. van der Graaf et al. (2007). "Levels of homocysteine are increased in metabolic syndrome patients but are not associated with an increased cardiovascular risk, in contrast to patients without the metabolic syndrome." *Heart* 93(2): 216–220.

Hajjar, K. (1993). "Homocysteine-induced modulation of tissue plasminogen activator binding to its endothelial cell membrane receptor." *J Clin Invest* 91: 2873–2879.

Halliwell, B. (1994). "Free radicals, antioxidants, and human disease: Curiosity, cause, or consequence?" *Lancet* 344: 721–724.

Hargrove, J. L., J. F. Trotter et al. (1989). "Experimental diabetes increases the formation of sulfane by transsulfuration and inactivation of tyrosine aminotransferase in cytosols from rat liver." *Metabolism* 38(7): 666–672.

Harpel, P., V. Chang et al. (1992). "Homocysteine and other sulfhydryl compounds enhance the binding of lipoprotein(a) to fibrin: A potential biochemical link between thrombosis, atherogenesis and sulfhydryl compound metabolism." *Proc Natl Acad Sci* 89: 10193–10197.

Harris, M. I. (1985). "Prevalence of noninsulin-dependent diabetes and impaired glucose tolerance. In: National Diabetes Data Group, eds. Diabetes in America: Diabetes data compiled 1984. U.S. Department of Health and Human Services publication (PHS) 85-1468." *National Institutes of Health* VI 1–31.32.

He, K., K. Liu et al. (2006). "Magnesium intake and incidence of metabolic syndrome among young adults." *Circulation* 113(13): 1675–1682.

Heinecke, J. W., M. Kawamura et al. (1993). "Oxidation of low density lipoprotein by thiols: Superoxide-dependent and -independent mechanisms." *J Lipid Res* 34(12): 2051–2061.

Hofmann, M. A., E. Lalla et al. (2001). "Hyperhomocysteinemia enhances vascular inflammation and accelerates atherosclerosis in a murine model." *J Clin Invest* 107(6): 675–683.

Holick, M. F. (2004). "Vitamin D: Importance in the prevention of cancers, type 1 diabetes, heart disease, and osteoporosis." *Am J Clin Nutr* 79(3): 362–371.

Holick, M. F. (2007). "Vitamin D deficiency." *N Engl J Med* 357(3): 266–281.

Hollis, B. W., J. Q. Kamerud et al. (1993). "Determination of vitamin D status by radioimmunoassay with an 125I-labeled tracer." *Clin Chem* 39(3): 529–533.

Hollis, B. W. and J. L. Napoli (1985). "Improved radioimmunoassay for vitamin D and its use in assessing vitamin D status." *Clin Chem* 31(11): 1815–1819.

Hoogeveen, E. K., P. J. Kostense et al. (2000). "Hyperhomocysteinemia increases risk of death, especially in type 2 diabetes: 5-year follow-up of the Hoorn Study." *Circulation* 101(13): 1506–1511.

Hotamisligil, G. S., N. S. Shargill et al. (1993). "Adipose expression of tumor necrosis factor-alpha: Direct role in obesity-linked insulin resistance." *Science* **259**(5091): 87–91.

House, J. D., R. L. Jacobs et al. (1999). "Regulation of homocysteine metabolism." *Adv Enzyme Regul* **39**: 69–91.

Humphries, S., H. Kushner et al. (1999). "Low dietary magnesium is associated with insulin resistance in a sample of young, nondiabetic black Americans." *Am J Hyperten* **12**: 747–756.

Hunter-Lavin, C., P. R. Hudson et al. (2004). "Folate supplementation reduces serum hsp70 levels in patients with type 2 diabetes." *Cell Stress Chaperones* **9**(4): 344–349.

Hypponen, E., B. J. Boucher et al. (2008). "25-hydroxyvitamin D, IGF-1, and metabolic syndrome at 45 years of age: A cross-sectional study in the 1958 British Birth Cohort." *Diabetes* **57**(2): 298–305.

Itoh, K., T. Kawasaka et al. (1997). "The effects of high oral magnesium supplementation on blood pressure, serum lipids and related variables in apparently healthy Japanese subjects." *Br J Nutr* **78**(5): 737–750.

Jain, S. K. and M. Palmer (1997). "The effect of oxygen radicals metabolites and vitamin E on glycosylation of proteins." *Free Radic Biol Med* **22**(4): 593–596.

Jee, S. H., E. R. Miller (2002). "The effect of magnesium supplementation on blood pressure: A meta-analysis of randomized clinical trials." *Am J Hypertens* **15**(8): 691–696.

Kadowaki, S. and A. W. Norman (1984). "Dietary vitamin D is essential for normal insulin secretion from the perfused rat pancreas." *J Clin Invest* **73**(3): 759–766.

Kahn, C. R. (1994). "Insulin action, diabetogenes, and the cause of type II diabetes." *Diabetes* **43**: 1066–1084.

Kang, S. S., P. W. K. Wong et al. (1987). "Homocysteinemia due to folate deficiency." *Metabolism* **36**: 458–462.

Kao, W. H., A. R. Folsom et al. (1999). "Serum and dietary magnesium and the risk for type 2 diabetes mellitus: The Atherosclerosis Risk in Communities Study." *Arch Intern Med* **159**(18): 2151–2159.

Karppanen, H., A. Tanskanen et al. (1984). "Safety and effects of potassium- and magnesium-containing low sodium salt mixtures." *J Cardiovasc Pharmacol* **6** (Suppl. 1): S236–243.

Kashiwagi, A., K. Shinozaki et al. (1999a). "Endothelium-specific activation of NAD(P)H oxidase in aortas of exogenously hyperinsulinemic rats." *Am J Physiol* **277**(6 Pt 1): E976–983.

Kashiwagi, A., K. Shinozaki et al. (1999b). "Free radical production in endothelial cells as a pathogenetic factor for vascular dysfunction in the insulin resistance state." *Diabetes Res Clin Pract* **45**(2–3): 199–203.

Kershaw, E. E. and J. S. Flier (2004). "Adipose tissue as an endocrine organ." *J Clin Endocrinol Metab* **89**(6): 2548–2556.

Kim, I., D. F. Williamson et al. (1993). "Vitamin and mineral supplement use and mortality in a US cohort." *Am J Public Health* **83**(4): 546–550.

Kim, J. A., M. Montagnani et al. (2006). "Reciprocal relationships between insulin resistance and endothelial dysfunction: Molecular and pathophysiological mechanisms." *Circulation* **113**(15): 1888–1904.

King, D. E., A. G. Mainous et al. (2005). "Dietary magnesium and C-reactive protein levels." *J Am Coll Nutr* **24**(3): 166–171.

Kirsten, R., B. Heintz et al. (1988). "Magnesium pyridoxal 5-phosphate glutamate reduces hyperlipidaemia in patients with chronic renal insufficiency." *Eur J Clin Pharmacol* **34**(2): 133–137.

Knekt, P., M. Laaksonen et al. (2008). "Serum vitamin D and subsequent occurrence of type 2 diabetes." *Epidemiology* **19**(5): 666–671.

Koh-Banerjee, P., M. Franz et al. (2004). "Changes in whole-grain, bran, and cereal fiber consumption in relation to 8-y weight gain among men." *Am J Clin Nutr* **80**(5): 1237–1245.

Kramer, J. H., I. T. Mak et al. (2003). "Dietary magnesium intake influences circulating pro-inflammatory neuropeptide levels and loss of myocardial tolerance to postischemic stress." *Exp Biol Med (Maywood)* **228**(6): 665–673.

Kritchevsky, S. B., A. J. Bush et al. (2000). "Serum carotenoids and markers of inflammation in nonsmokers." *Am J Epidemiol* **152**(11): 1065–1071.

Kurantsin-Mills, J., M. M. Cassidy et al. (1997). "Marked alterations in circulating inflammatory cells during cardiomyopathy development in a magnesium-deficient rat model." *Br J Nutr* **78**(5): 845–855.

Labadarios, D., P. A. Brink et al. (1987). "Plasma vitamin A, E, C and B6 levels in myocardial infarction." *S Afr Med J* **71**(9): 561–563.

Larsson, S. C., L. Bergkvist et al. (2005). "Magnesium intake in relation to risk of colorectal cancer in women." *JAMA* **293**(1): 86–89.

Larsson, S. C. and A. Wolk (2007). "Magnesium intake and risk of type 2 diabetes: A meta-analysis." *J Intern Med* **262**(2): 208–214.

LeBoff, M. S., L. Kohlmeier et al. (1999). "Occult vitamin D deficiency in postmenopausal US women with acute hip fracture." *JAMA* **281**(16): 1505–1511.

Lentz, S. and J. Sadler (1991). "Inhibition of thrombomodulin surface expression and protein C activation by the thrombogenic agent homocysteine." *J Clin Invest* **88**: 1906–1914.

Lerner, M. (1998). "Vitamin E markets bullish, boosting capacity and price." *Chem Market Report* **253**: 18–19.

Levin, G., H. Mather et al. (1981). "Tissue magnesium status in diabetes mellitus." *Diabetologia* **21**: 131–134.

Li, G., P. Zhang et al. (2008). "The long-term effect of lifestyle interventions to prevent diabetes in the China Da Qing Diabetes Prevention Study: A 20-year follow-up study. *Lancet* **371**(9626): 1783–1789.

Liao, F., A. R. Folsom et al. (1998). "Is low magnesium concentration a risk factor for coronary heart disease? The Atherosclerosis Risk in Communities (ARIC) Study." *Am Heart J* **136**(3): 480–490.

Lindebaum, J., I. Rosenburg et al. (1994). "Prevalence of cobalamin deficiency in the Framingham elderly population." *Am J Clin Nutr* **60**: 2–11.

Liu, E., J. B. Meigs et al. (2009). "Plasma 25-hydroxyvitamin D is associated with markers of the insulin resistant phenotype in nondiabetic adults." *J Nutr* **139**(2): 329–334.

Liu, S., H. K. Choi et al. (2006). "A prospective study of dairy intake and the risk of type 2 diabetes in women." *Diabetes Care* **29**(7): 1579–1584.

Liu, S., I. M. Lee et al. (2006). "Vitamin E and risk of type 2 diabetes in the women's health study randomized controlled trial." *Diabetes* **55**(10): 2856–2862.

Liu, S., J. E. Manson et al. (2000). "A prospective study of whole-grain intake and risk of type 2 diabetes mellitus in US women." *Am J Public Health* **90**(9): 1409–1415.

Liu, S., Y. Song et al. (2005). "Dietary calcium, vitamin D, and the prevalence of metabolic syndrome in middle-aged and older U.S. women." *Diabetes Care* **28**(12): 2926–2932.

Liu, S., W. C. Willett et al. (2003). "Relation between changes in intakes of dietary fiber and grain products and changes in weight and development of obesity among middle-aged women." *Am J Clin Nutr* **78**(5): 920–927.

Loscalzo, J. (1996). "The oxidant stress of hyperhomocyst(e)inemia." *J Clin Invest* **98**(1): 5–7.

Louw, J. A., A. Werbeck et al. (1992). "Blood vitamin concentrations during the acute-phase response." *Crit Care Med* **20**(7): 934–941.

Lyons, T. J. (1992). "Lipoprotein glycation and its metabolic consequences." *Diabetes* **41 Suppl 2**(4): 67–73.

Ma, J., A. R. Folsom et al. (1995). "Associations of serum and dietary magnesium with cardiovascular disease, hypertension, diabetes, insulin, and carotid arterial wall thickness: The ARIC study. Atherosclerosis Risk in Communities Study." *J Clin Epidemiol* **48**(7): 927–940.

MacLaughlin, J. and M. F. Holick (1985). "Aging decreases the capacity of human skin to produce vitamin D3." *J Clin Invest* **76**(4): 1536–1538.

Malabanan, A., I. E. Veronikis et al. (1998). "Redefining vitamin D insufficiency." *Lancet* **351**(9105): 805–806.

Malecki, M. T., J. Frey et al. (2003). "Vitamin D receptor gene polymorphisms and association with type 2 diabetes mellitus in a Polish population." *Exp Clin Endocrinol Diabetes* **111**(8): 505–509.

Mangoni, A. A., R. A. Sherwood et al. (2005). "Short-term oral folic acid supplementation enhances endothelial function in patients with type 2 diabetes." *Am J Hypertens* **18**(2 Pt 1): 220–226.

Manolio, T. A., P. J. Savage et al. (1991). "Correlates of fasting insulin levels in young adults: The CARDIA study." *J Clin Epidemiol* **44**(6): 571–578.

Manson, J. and A. Spelsberg (1994). "Primary prevention of non-insulin-dependent diabetes mellitus." *Am J Prev Med* **10**: 172–184.

Marken, P. A., C. W. Weart et al. (1989). "Effects of magnesium oxide on the lipid profile of healthy volunteers." *Atherosclerosis* **77**(1): 37–42.

Massy, Z. A. (2000). "Importance of homocysteine, lipoprotein (a) and non-classical cardiovascular risk factors (fibrinogen and advanced glycation end-products) for atherogenesis in uraemic patients." *Nephrol Dial Transplant* **15**(Suppl 5): 81–91.

Massy, Z. A., Y. Kim et al. (2000). "Low-density lipoprotein-induced expression of interleukin-6, a marker of human mesangial cell inflammation: Effects of oxidation and modulation by lovastatin." *Biochem Biophys Res Commun* **267**(2): 536–540.

Mather, H., J. A. Nisbet et al. (1979). "Hypomagnesemia in diabetes." *Clin Chim Acta* **95**: 235–242.

Mathieu, C., C. Gysemans et al. (2005). "Vitamin D and diabetes." *Diabetologia* **48**(7): 1247–1257.

Mattila, C., P. Knekt et al. (2007). "Serum 25-hydroxyvitamin D concentration and subsequent risk of type 2 diabetes." *Diabetes Care* **30**(10): 2569–2570.

McCully, K. S. (1969). "Vascular pathology of homocysteinemia: Implications for the pathogenesis of arteriosclerosis." *Am J Pathol* **56**(1): 111–128.

McDonald, J. (1986). "Vitamin and mineral supplement use in the United States." *Clin Nutr* **5**: 27–33.

McKeown, N. M., J. B. Meigs et al. (2004). "Carbohydrate nutrition, insulin resistance, and the prevalence of the metabolic syndrome in the Framingham Offspring Cohort." _Diabetes Care_ 27(2): 538–546.

McMillan, D. C., N. Sattar et al. (2000). "Changes in micronutrient concentrations following anti-inflammatory treatment in patients with gastrointestinal cancer." _Nutrition_ 16(6): 425–428.

McNair, P., M. S. Christensen et al. (1982). "Renal hypomagnesaemia in human diabetes mellitus: Its relation to glucose homeostasis." _Eur J Clin Invest_ 12(1): 81–85.

Meigs, J. B., P. F. Jacques et al. (2001). "Fasting plasma homocysteine levels in the insulin resistance syndrome: The Framingham offspring study." _Diabetes Care_ 24(8): 1403–1410.

Meyer, K. A., L. H. Kushi et al. (2000). "Carbohydrates, dietary fiber, and incident type 2 diabetes in older women." _Am J Clin Nutr_ 71(4): 921–930.

Michaud, D. S., E. L. Giovannucci et al. (1998). "Associations of plasma carotenoid concentrations and dietary intake of specific carotenoids in samples of two prospective cohort studies using a new carotenoid database." _Cancer Epidemiol Biomarkers Prev_ 7: 283–290.

Milner, R. D. and C. N. Hales (1967). "The role of calcium and magnesium in insulin secretion from rabbit pancreas studied in vitro." _Diabetologia_ 3(1): 47–49.

Mizushima, S., F. P. Cappuccio et al. (1998). "Dietary magnesium intake and blood pressure: A qualitative overview of the observational studies." _J Hum Hypertens_ 12(7): 447–453.

Mohamed-Ali, V., J. H. Pinkney et al. (1998). "Adipose tissue as an endocrine and paracrine organ." _Int J Obes Relat Metab Disord_ 22(12): 1145–1158.

Mullan, B. A., I. S. Young et al. (2002). "Ascorbic acid reduces blood pressure and arterial stiffness in type 2 diabetes." _Hypertension_ 40(6): 804–809.

Munshi, M. N., A. Stone et al. (1996). "Hyperhomocysteinemia following a methionine load in patients with non-insulin-dependent diabetes mellitus and macrovascular disease." _Metabolism_ 45(1): 133–135.

Nadler, J. L., T. Buchanan et al. (1993). "Magnesium deficiency produces insulin resistance and increased thromboxan synthesis." _Hypertension_ 21: 1024–1029.

Nagpal, J., J. N. Pande et al. (2009). "A double-blind, randomized, placebo-controlled trial of the short-term effect of vitamin D3 supplementation on insulin sensitivity in apparently healthy, middle-aged, centrally obese men." _Diabet Med_ 26(1): 19–27.

Nappo, F., N. De Rosa et al. (1999). "Impairment of endothelial functions by acute hyperhomocysteinemia and reversal by antioxidant vitamins." _JAMA_ 281(22): 2113–2118.

Nathan, D. M., D. S. S.

NCEP (2001). "Executive Summary of The Third Report of The National Cholesterol Education Program (NCEP) Expert Panel on Detection, Evaluation, And Treatment of High Blood Cholesterol In Adults (Adult Treatment Panel III)." _JAMA_ 285(19): 2486–2497.

Need, A. G., H. A. Morris et al. (1993). "Effects of skin thickness, age, body fat, and sunlight on serum 25-hydroxyvitamin D." _Am J Clin Nutr_ 58(6): 882–885.

Need, A. G., P. D. O'Loughlin et al. (2005). "Relationship between fasting serum glucose, age, body mass index and serum 25 hydroxyvitamin D in postmenopausal women." _Clin Endocrinol (Oxf)_ 62(6): 738–741.

NIH (2006). "National Institutes of Health State-of-the-science conference statement: Multivitamin/mineral supplements and chronic disease prevention." *Ann Intern Med* **145**(5): 364–371.

Norman, A. W. (2008). "From vitamin D to hormone D: Fundamentals of the vitamin D endocrine system essential for good health." *Am J Clin Nutr* **88**(2): 491S–499S.

Norman, A. W., J. B. Frankel et al. (1980). "Vitamin D deficiency inhibits pancreatic secretion of insulin." *Science* **209**(4458): 823–825.

Nyomba, B. L., R. Bouillon et al. (1984). "Influence of vitamin D status on insulin secretion and glucose tolerance in the rabbit." *Endocrinology* **115**(1): 191–197.

O'Keefe, C. A., L. B. Bailey et al. (1995). "Controlled dietary folate affects folate status in nonpregnant women." *J Nutr* **125**: 2717–2725.

Oberley, L. W. (1988). "Free radicals and diabetes." *Free Radic Biol Med* **5**(2): 113–124.

Ogunkolade, B. W., B. J. Boucher et al. (2002). "Vitamin D receptor (VDR) mRNA and VDR protein levels in relation to vitamin D status, insulin secretory capacity, and VDR genotype in Bangladeshi Asians." *Diabetes* **51**(7): 2294–2300.

Oh, J. Y. and E. Barrett-Connor (2002). "Association between vitamin D receptor polymorphism and type 2 diabetes or metabolic syndrome in community-dwelling older adults: The Rancho Bernardo Study." *Metabolism* **51**(3): 356–359.

Ortlepp, J. R., J. Metrikat et al. (2003). "The vitamin D receptor gene variant and physical activity predicts fasting glucose levels in healthy young men." *Diabet Med* **20**(6): 451–454.

Orwoll, E., M. Riddle et al. (1994). "Effects of vitamin D on insulin and glucagon secretion in non-insulin-dependent diabetes mellitus." *Am J Clin Nutr* **59**(5): 1083–1087.

Packer, L. (1991). "Protective role of vitamin E in biological systems." *Am J Clin Nutr* **53**: 1050S–1055S.

Padayatty, S. J., A. Katz et al. (2003). "Vitamin C as an antioxidant: Evaluation of its role in disease prevention." *J Am Coll Nutr* **22**(1): 18–35.

Palomer, X., J. M. Gonzalez-Clemente et al. (2008). "Role of vitamin D in the pathogenesis of type 2 diabetes mellitus." *Diabetes Obes Metab* **10**(3): 185–197.

Pan, X., H. Cao et al. (1997). "Effects of diet and exercise in preventing NIDDM in people with impaired glucose tolerance." *Diabetes care* **20**: 537–544.

Paolisso, D., A. D'Amore et al. (1993). "Pharmacologic doses of vitamin E improve insulin action in healthy subjects and non-insulin-dependent diabetic patients." *Am J Clin Nutr* **57**: 650–656.

Paolisso, G., V. Balbi et al. (1995). "Metabolic benefits deriving from chronic vitamin C supplementation in aged non-insulin dependent diabetics." *J Am Coll Nutr* **14**(4): 387–392.

Paolisso, G. and M. Barbagallo (1997). "Hypertension, diabetes mellitus, and insulin resistance: The role of intracellular magnesium." *Am J Hypertens* **10**: 346–355.

Paolisso, G., A. D'Amore et al. (1993). "Evidence for a relationship between free radicals and insulin action in the elderly." *Metabolism* **42**: 659–663.

Paolisso, G. and D. Giugliano (1996). "Oxidative stress and insulin action: Is there a relationship?" *Diabetologia* **39**(3): 357–363.

Paolisso, G., D. Giugliano et al. (1992). "Glutathione infusion potentiates glucose-induced insulin secretion in aged patients with impaired glucose tolerance." *Diabetes Care* **15**(1): 1–7.

Paolisso, G. and E. Ravusin (1995). "Intracellular magnesium and insulin resistance: Results in Pima Indians and Caucasians." *J Clin Endocrinol Metab.* **80**: 1382–1385.

Paolisso, G., A. Scheen et al. (1994). "Changes in glucose turnover parameters and improvement of glucose oxidation after 4-week magnesium administration in elderly noninsulin-dependent (type II) diabetic patients." *J Clin Endocrinol Metab* **78**(6): 1510–1514.

Paolisso, G., A. Scheen et al. (1990). "Magnesium and glucose homeostasis." *Diabetologia* **33**(9): 511–514.

Paolisso, G., S. Sgambato et al. (1992). "Daily magnesium supplements improve glucose handling in elderly subjects." *Am J Clin Nutr* **55**(6): 1161–1167.

Paolisso, G., S. Sgambato et al. (1989). "Improved insulin response and action by chronic magnesium administration in aged NIDDM subjects." *Diabetes Care* **12**(4): 265–269.

Parasarathy, S. (1987). "Oxidation of low density lipoprotein by thiol compounds leads to its recognition by the acetyl LDL receptor." *Biochem Biophys Acta* **917**: 3337–3340.

Passaro, A., K. D'Elia et al. (2000). "Factors influencing plasma homocysteine levels in type 2 diabetes [letter]." *Diabetes Care* **23**(3): 420–421.

Peacock, J. M., A. R. Folsom et al. (1999). "Relationship of serum and dietary magnesium to incident hypertension: The Atherosclerosis Risk in Communities (ARIC) Study." *Ann Epidemiol* **9**(3): 159–165.

Pearson, P. J., P. R. Evora et al. (1998). "Hypomagnesemia inhibits nitric oxide release from coronary endothelium: Protective role of magnesium infusion after cardiac operations." *Ann Thorac Surg* **65**(4): 967–972.

Penckofer, S., J. Kouba et al. (2008). "Vitamin D and diabetes: Let the sunshine in." *Diabetes Educ* **34**(6): 939–940, 942, 944 passim.

Pennington, J. A. T. and B. E. Young (1991). "Total Diet Study: Nutritional elements." *J Am Diet Assoc* **91**: 179.

Petitti, D. B. (2000). *Meta-Analysis, Decision Analysis, and Cost-Effectiveness Analysis.* NewYork, Oxford University Press, Inc.

Pinkney, J. H., C. D. Stehouwer et al. (1997). "Endothelial dysfunction: Cause of the insulin resistance syndrome." *Diabetes* **46**(Suppl. 2): S9–13.

Pittas, A. G., B. Dawson-Hughes et al. (2006). "Vitamin D and calcium intake in relation to type 2 diabetes in women." *Diabetes Care* **29**(3): 650–656.

Pittas, A. G., S. S. Harris et al. (2007). "The effects of calcium and vitamin D supplementation on blood glucose and markers of inflammation in nondiabetic adults." *Diabetes Care* **30**(4): 980–986.

Pittas, A. G., J. Lau et al. (2007). "The role of vitamin D and calcium in type 2 diabetes: A systematic review and meta-analysis." *J Clin Endocrinol Metab* **92**(6): 2017–2029.

Price, D. T. and J. Loscalzo (1999). "Cellular adhesion molecules and atherogenesis." *Am J Med* **107**(1): 85–97.

Purvis, J. R., D. M. Cummings et al. (1994). "Effect of oral magnesium supplementation on selected cardiovascular risk factors in non-insulin-dependent diabetics." *Arch Fam Med* **3**(6): 503–508.

Pyorala, K. (1979). "Relationship of glucose tolerance and plasma insulin to the incidence of coronary heart disease: Results from two population studies in Finland." *Diabetes Care* **2**: 131–141.

Rasmussen, H. S., P. Aurup et al. (1989). "Influence of magnesium substitution therapy on blood lipid composition in patients with ischemic heart disease: A double-blind, placebo controlled study." *Arch Intern Med* **149**(5): 1050–1053.

Rayssiguier, Y. (1984). "Role of magnesium and potassium in the pathogenesis of arteriosclerosis." *Magnesium* **3**(4–6): 226–238.

Rayssiguier, Y., E. Gueux et al. (1981). "Effect of magnesium deficiency on lipid metabolism in rats fed a high carbohydrate diet." *J Nutr* **111**(11): 1876–1883.

Rayssiguier, Y., L. Noe et al. (1991). "Effect of magnesium deficiency on postheparin lipase activity and tissue lipoprotein lipase in the rat." *Lipids* **26**(3): 182–186.

Regensteiner, J. G., S. Popylisen et al. (2003). "Oral L-arginine and vitamins E and C improve endothelial function in women with type 2 diabetes." *Vasc Med* **8**(3): 169–175.

Reinhart, R. A. (1988). "Magnesium metabolism. A review with special reference to the relationship between intracellular content and serum levels." *Arch Intern Med* **148**(11): 2415–2420.

Resnick, L., B. T. Altura et al. (1993). "Intracellular and extracellular magnesium depletion in type 2 diabetes mellitus." *Diabetologia* **36**: 767–770.

Reunanen, A., P. Knekt et al. (1998). "Serum antioxidants and risk of non-insulin dependent diabetes mellitus." *Eur J Clin Nutr* **52**(2): 89–93.

Rivett, A. J. (1985a). "Preferential degradation of the oxidatively modified form of glutamine synthetase by intracellular mammalian proteases." *J Biol Chem* **260**(1): 300–305.

Rivett, A. J. (1985b). "Purification of a liver alkaline protease which degrades oxidatively modified glutamine synthetase: Characterization as a high molecular weight cysteine proteinase." *J Biol Chem* **260**(23): 12600–12606.

Robillon, J. F., B. Canivet et al. (1994). "Type 1 diabetes mellitus and homocyst(e)ine." *Diabete Metab* **20**(5): 494–496.

Rock, C., M. Jahnke et al. (1997). "Racial group differences in plasma concentrations of antioxidant vitamins and carotenoids in hemodialysis patients." *Am J Clin Nutr* **65**: 844–850.

Rock, C. L. (2007). "Multivitamin-multimineral supplements: Who uses them?" *Am J Clin Nutr* **85**(1): 277S–279S.

Rodriguez-Moran, M. and F. Guerrero-Romero (2003). "Oral magnesium supplementation improves insulin sensitivity and metabolic control in type 2 diabetic subjects: A randomized double-blind controlled trial." *Diabetes Care* **26**(4): 1147–1152.

Rosolova, H., O. Mayer et al. (1997). "Effect of variations in plasma magnesium concentration on resistance to insulin-mediated glucose disposal in nondiabetic subjects." *J Clin Endocrinol Metab* **82**: 3783–3785.

Rosolova, H., O. Mayer et al. (2000). "Insulin-mediated glucose disposal is decreased in normal subjects with relatively low plasma magnesium concentrations." *Metabolism* **49**: 418–420.

Saad, M., W. Knowler et al. (1988). "The natural history of impaired glucose tolerance in Pima Indians." *N Eng J Med* **319**: 1500–1506.

Salmeron, J., A. Ascherio et al. (1997). "Dietary fiber, glycemic load, and risk of NIDDM in men." *Diabetes Care* **20**(4): 545–550.

Salmeron, J., J. E. Manson et al. (1997). "Dietary fiber, glycemic load, and risk of non-insulin-dependent diabetes mellitus in women." *JAMA* **277**(6): 472–477.

Salonen, J. T., K. Nyyssonen et al. (1995). "Increased risk of non-insulin dependent diabetes mellitus at low plasma vitamin E concentrations: A four year follow up study in men." *BMJ* **311**(7013): 1124–1127.

Sargeant, L. A., N. J. Wareham et al. (2000). "Vitamin C and hyperglycemia in the European Prospective Investigation into Cancer—Norfolk (EPIC-Norfolk) study: A population-based study." *Diabetes Care* **23**(6): 726–732.

Saris, N. E., E. Mervaala et al. (2000). "Magnesium. An update on physiological, clinical and analytical aspects." *Clin Chim Acta* **294**(1–2): 1–26.

Schmidt, L. E., C. L. Arfken et al. (1994). "Evaluation of nutrient intake in subjects with non-insulin-dependent diabetes mellitus." *J Am Diet Assoc* **94**(7): 773–774.

Schram, M. T. and C. D. Stehouwer (2005). "Endothelial dysfunction, cellular adhesion molecules and the metabolic syndrome." *Horm Metab Res* **37**(Suppl. 1): 49–55.

Schulze, M. B., M. Schulz et al. (2007). "Fiber and magnesium intake and incidence of type 2 diabetes: A prospective study and meta-analysis." *Arch Intern Med* **167**(9): 956–965.

Scragg, R., I. Holdaway et al. (1995). "Serum 25-hydroxyvitamin D3 levels decreased in impaired glucose tolerance and diabetes mellitus." *Diabetes Res Clin Pract* **27**(3): 181–188.

Scragg, R., M. Sowers et al. (2004). "Serum 25-hydroxyvitamin D, diabetes, and ethnicity in the Third National Health and Nutrition Examination Survey." *Diabetes Care* **27**(12): 2813–2818.

Seelig, M. S. and H. A. Heggtveit (1974). "Magnesium interrelationships in ischemic heart disease: A review." *Am J Clin Nutr* **27**(1): 59–79.

Selhub, J., P. F. Jacques et al. (1993). "Vitamin status and intake as primary determinants of homocysteinemia in an elderly population." *J Am Med Assoc* **270**: 2693–2698.

Shechter, M., M. Sharir et al. (2000). "Oral magnesium therapy improves endothelial function in patients with coronary artery disease." *Circulation* **102**(19): 2353–2358.

Sheu, W. H., W. J. Lee et al. (2000). "Plasma homocysteine concentrations and insulin sensitivity in hypertensive subjects." *Am J Hypertens* **13**(1 Pt 1): 14–20.

Sicree, R., P. Zimmet et al. (1987). "Plasma insulin response among Nauruans: Prediction of deterioration in glucose tolerance over 6 yr." *Diabetes* **36**: 179–186.

Sjogren, A., C. H. Floren et al. (1988a). "Magnesium, potassium and zinc deficiency in subjects with type II diabetes mellitus." *Acta Med Scand* **224**(5): 461–466.

Sjogren, A., C. H. Floren et al. (1988b). "Oral administration of magnesium hydroxide to subjects with insulin-dependent diabetes mellitus: Effects on magnesium and potassium levels and on insulin requirements." *Magnesium* **7**(3): 117–122.

Smolin, L. and N. Benevenga (1982). "Accumulation of homocysteinemia in vitamin B6 deficiency." *J Nutr* **112**: 1264–1272.

Snijder, M. B., R. M. van Dam et al. (2005). "Adiposity in relation to vitamin D status and parathyroid hormone levels: A population-based study in older men and women." *J Clin Endocrinol Metab* **90**(7): 4119–4123.

Snijder, M. B., A. A. van der Heijden et al. (2007). "Is higher dairy consumption associated with lower body weight and fewer metabolic disturbances? The Hoorn Study." *Am J Clin Nutr* **85**(4): 989–995.

Snowdon, D. A. and R. L. Phillips (1985). "Does a vegetarian diet reduce the occurrence of diabetes?" *Am J Public Health* **75**: 509–512.

Sone, T., S. J. Marx et al. (1990). "A unique point mutation in the human vitamin D receptor chromosomal gene confers hereditary resistance to 1,25-dihydroxyvitamin D3." *Mol Endocrinol* **4**(4): 623–631.

Song, Y., N. R. Cook et al. (2009a). "Effect of homocysteine-lowering treatment with folic Acid and B vitamins on risk of type 2 diabetes in women: A randomized, controlled trial." *Diabetes* **58**(8): 1921–1928.

Song, Y., N. R. Cook et al. (2009b). "Effects of vitamins C and E and beta-carotene on the risk of type 2 diabetes in women at high risk of cardiovascular disease: A randomized controlled trial." *Am J Clin Nutr* **90**(2): 429–437.

Song, Y., E. S. Ford et al. (2005). "Relations of magnesium intake with metabolic risk factors and risks of type 2 diabetes, hypertension, and cardiovascular disease: A critical appraisal." *Curr Nut & Food Sci* **1**(3): 231–243.

Song, Y., T. Y. Li et al. (2007). "Magnesium intake and plasma concentrations of markers of systemic inflammation and endothelial dysfunction in women." *Am J Clin Nutr* **85**(4): 1068–1074.

Song, Y., J. E. Manson et al. (2004). "Dietary magnesium intake in relation to plasma insulin levels and risk of type 2 diabetes in women." *Diabetes Care* **27**(1): 59–65.

Song, Y., J. E. Manson et al. (2005). "Dietary magnesium intake and risk of cardiovascular disease among women." *Am J Cardiol* **96**(8): 1135–1141.

Song, Y., P. M. Ridker et al. (2005). "Magnesium intake, C-reactive protein, and the prevalence of metabolic syndrome in middle-aged and older U.S. women." *Diabetes Care* **28**(6): 1438–1444.

Song, Y., H. D. Sesso et al. (2006). "Dietary magnesium intake and risk of incident hypertension among middle-aged and older US women in a 10-year follow-up study." *Am J Cardiol* **98**: 1616–1621.

Song, Y., Q. Xu et al. (2011). "Multivitamins, individual vitamin and mineral supplements, and risk of diabetes among older U.S. adults." *Diabetes Care* **34**(1): 108–114.

Spoelstra-de, M. A., C. B. Brouwer et al. (2004). "No effect of folic acid on markers of endothelial dysfunction or inflammation in patients with type 2 diabetes mellitus and mild hyperhomocysteinaemia." *Neth J Med* **62**(7): 246–253.

Stamler, J. S., J. A. Osborne et al. (1993). "Adverse vascular effects of homocysteine are modulated by endothelium-derived relaxing factor and related oxides of nitrogen." *J Clin Invest* **91**(1): 308–318.

Stampfer, M. J., M. R. Malinow et al. (1992). "A prospective study of plasma homocyste(e)ine and risk of myocardial infarction in US physicians." *J Am Med Assoc* **268**: 877–881.

Starkebaum, G. and J. M. Harlan (1986). "Endothelial cell injury due to copper-catalyzed hydrogen peroxide generation from homocysteine." *J Clin Invest* **77**(4): 1370–1376.

Steinberg, D. (1991). "Antioxidants and atherosclerosis. A current assessment." *Circulation* **84**: 1420–1425.

Stern, M. P. (1995). "Diabetes and cardiovascular disease: The 'common soil' hypothesis." *Diabetes* **44**: 369–374.

Stitt, F. W., D. G. Clayton et al. (1973). "Clinical and biochemical indicators of cardiovascular disease among men living in hard and soft water areas." *Lancet* **1**(7795): 122–126.

Stout, R. W. (1990). "Insulin and atheroma. 20-yr perspective." *Diabetes Care* **13**(6): 631–654.

Suarez, A., N. Pulido et al. (1995). "Impaired tyrosine-kinase activity of muscle insulin receptors from hypomagnesaemic rats." *Diabetologia* **38**: 1262–1270.

Tai, K., A. G. Need et al. (2008). "Vitamin D, glucose, insulin, and insulin sensitivity." *Nutrition* **24**(3): 279–285.

Talwar, D., T. K. Ha et al. (1997). "Effect of inflammation on measures of antioxidant status in patients with non-small cell lung cancer." *Am J Clin Nutr* **66**(5): 1283–1285.

Title, L. M., E. Ur et al. (2006). "Folic acid improves endothelial dysfunction in type 2 diabetes—an effect independent of homocysteine-lowering." *Vasc Med* **11**(2): 101–109.

Touyz, R. M. (2003). "Role of magnesium in the pathogenesis of hypertension." *Mol Aspects Med* **24**(1–3): 107–136.

Touyz, R. M. (2004). "Magnesium in clinical medicine." *Front Biosci* **9**: 1278–1293.

Tucker, K. L., B. Mahnken et al. (1996). "Folic acid fortification of the food supply: Potential benefits and risks for the elderly population." *J Am Med Assoc* **276**: 1879–1885.

Ubbink, J. B., W. J. H. Vermaak et al. (1994). "Vitamin requirements for the treatment of hyperhomocysteinemia in humans." *J Nutr* **124**: 1927–1933.

Upritchard, J. E., W. H. Sutherland et al. (2000). "Effect of supplementation with tomato juice, vitamin E, and vitamin C on LDL oxidation and products of inflammatory activity in type 2 diabetes." *Diabetes Care* **23**(6): 733–738.

Uysal, K. T., S. M. Wiesbrock et al. (1997). "Protection from obesity-induced insulin resistance in mice lacking TNF-alpha function." *Nature* **389**(6651): 610–614.

van Dam, R. M., F. B. Hu et al. (2006). "Dietary calcium and magnesium, major food sources, and risk of type 2 diabetes in U.S. black women." *Diabetes Care* **29**(10): 2238–2243.

van Etten, R. W., E. J. de Koning et al. (2002). "Impaired NO-dependent vasodilation in patients with Type II (non-insulin-dependent) diabetes mellitus is restored by acute administration of folate." *Diabetologia* **45**(7): 1004–1010.

van Guldener, C. and C. D. Stehouwer (2002). "Diabetes mellitus and hyperhomocysteinemia." *Semin Vasc Med* **2**(1): 87–95.

van het Hof, K. H., I. A. Brouwer et al. (1999). "Bioavailability of lutein from vegetables is 5 times higher than that of beta-carotene." *Am J Clin Nutr* **70**(2): 261–268.

Vaquero, M. P. (2002). "Magnesium and trace elements in the elderly: Intake, status and recommendations." *J Nutr Health Aging* **6**(2): 147–153.

Vitale, J. J., P. L. White et al. (1957). "Interrelationships between experimental hypercholesteremia, magnesium requirement, and experimental atherosclerosis." *J Exp Med* **106**(5): 757–766.

Wajchenberg, B. L. (2000). "Subcutaneous and visceral adipose tissue: Their relation to the metabolic syndrome." *Endocr Rev* **21**(6): 697–738.

Wang, X., X. Qin et al. (2007). "Efficacy of folic acid supplementation in stroke prevention: A meta-analysis." *Lancet* **369**(9576): 1876–1882.

Weglicki, W. B., B. F. Dickens et al. (1996). "Immunoregulation by neuropeptides in magnesium deficiency: Ex vivo effect of enhanced substance P production on circulating T lymphocytes from magnesium-deficient mice." *Magnes Res* **9**(1): 3–11.

Weglicki, W. B., T. M. Phillips et al. (1992). "Magnesium-deficiency elevates circulating levels of inflammatory cytokines and endothelin." *Mol Cell Biochem* **110**(2): 169–173.

Weiss, N., S. J. Heydrick et al. (2003). "Influence of hyperhomocysteinemia on the cellular redox state— impact on homocysteine-induced endothelial dysfunction." *Clin Chem Lab Med* **41**(11): 1455–1461.

Welch, G. N. and J. Loscalzo (1998). "Homocysteine and atherothrombosis." *N Engl J Med* **338**(15): 1042–1050.

Wells, W. W., C. Z. Dou et al. (1995). "Ascorbic acid is essential for the release of insulin from scorbutic guinea pig pancreatic islets." *Proc Natl Acad Sci U S A* **92**(25): 11869–11873.

Whelton, P. and M. Klag (1989).

Will, J. C. and T. Byers (1996). "Does diabetes mellitus increase the requirement for vitamin C?" *Nutr Rev* **54**: 193–202.

Willett, W. C. (1998). *Nutritional Epidemiology, Second Edition*. New York, Oxford University Press.

Williamson, J. R., K. Chang et al. (1993). "Hyperglycemic pseudohypoxia and diabetic complications." *Diabetes* **42**(6): 801–813.

Wilson, P. W. and S. M. Grundy (2003a). "The metabolic syndrome: A practical guide to origins and treatment: Part II." *Circulation* **108**(13): 1537–1540.

Wilson, P. W. and S. M. Grundy (2003b). "The metabolic syndrome: Practical guide to origins and treatment: Part I." *Circulation* **108**(12): 1422–1424.

Wilson, P. W. and W. B. Kannel (2002). "Obesity, diabetes, and risk of cardiovascular disease in the elderly." *Am J Geriatr Cardiol* **11**(2): 119–123, 125.

Witteman, J. C., W. C. Willett et al. (1989). "A prospective study of nutritional factors and hypertension among US women." *Circulation* **80**(5): 1320–1327.

Xu, L. and M. Z. Badr (1999). "Enhanced potential for oxidative stress in hyperinsulinemic rats: Imbalance between hepatic peroxisomal hydrogen peroxide production and decomposition due to hyperinsulinemia." *Horm Metab Res* **31**(4): 278–282.

Xu, Q., C. G. Parks et al. (2009). "Multivitamin use and telomere length in women." *Am J Clin Nutr* **89**(6): 1857–1863.

Yajnik, C. S., R. F. Smith et al. (1984). "Fasting plasma magnesium concentrations and glucose disposal in diabetes." *Br Med J (Clin Res Ed)* **288**(6423): 1032–1034.

Yamori, Y. and S. Mizushima (2000). "A reiview of the link between dietary magnesium and cardiovascular risk." *J Cardiovasc Risk* **7**: 31–35.

Ye, W. Z., A. F. Reis et al. (2001). "Vitamin D receptor gene polymorphisms are associated with obesity in type 2 diabetic subjects with early age of onset." *Eur J Endocrinol* **145**(2): 181–186.

Yokota, K., M. Kato et al. (2004). "Clinical efficacy of magnesium supplementation in patients with type 2 diabetes." *J Am Coll Nutr* **23**(5): 506S–509S.

Zeisel, S. (1999). "Regulation of 'Nutraceuticals.'" *Science* **285**: 1853–1854.

Zeitz, U., K. Weber et al. (2003). "Impaired insulin secretory capacity in mice lacking a functional vitamin D receptor." *Faseb J* **17**(3): 509–511.

Zittermann, A., S. Frisch et al. (2009). "Vitamin D supplementation enhances the beneficial effects of weight loss on cardiovascular disease risk markers." *Am J Clin Nutr* **89**(5): 1321–1327.

chapter six

Dietary patterns and type 2 diabetes

Andrew O. Odegaard, PhD

Mark A. Pereira, PhD
University of Minnesota

Contents

Historical evidence demonstrates a fundamental role for dietary intake in the etiology and prevention of type 2 diabetes, and thus the global type 2 diabetes epidemic. As outlined throughout this book, the evidence base for understanding dietary intake and type 2 diabetes is extensive and growing. With this expanding foundation of knowledge it is human nature to reduce and simplify. Alternatively, there is a need to recognize the inherent complexity of dietary intake with its scores of constituents and considerations. And it is here, where dietary patterns research has developed as a tool to understanding the complicated diet–diabetes relationship. Indeed, across populations, dietary patterns have emerged sharing consistencies and many characteristics relative to etiology and prevention of type 2 diabetes. These patterns are especially significant when one considers that an overall pattern exerts itself pleiotropically on numerous pathways relevant to the etiology of type 2 diabetes, including energy balance, insulin resistance/sensitivity, glycemia, inflammation, endothelial function, etc. This chapter discusses the essential role of dietary patterns in relation to type 2 diabetes.

Rationale for studying dietary patterns

There are both conceptual and methodological grounds for studying dietary patterns in nutrition research, both stemming from the core axiom that populations and the people that comprise them eat a diet with many constituents, often consumed together, in characteristic patterns. Hence, from a conceptual standpoint studying dietary patterns in relation to diabetes is appealing because they encapsulate usual habits and how people actually eat in variety and frequency (McKeown and Jacobs, 2010). This approach provides an attractive paradigm for investigation in large epidemiological studies, and to serve as the main basis for dietary recommendations for prevention.

Despite the complexity of dietary intake, historical approaches to studying diet–diabetes relationships have focused on a reductionist approach examining single nutrients or foods with the disease. This precedent likely stems from the original efforts of the USDA of setting nutrient targets for dietary recommendations (Mozaffarian and Ludwig, 2010; Nestle, 2002), statistical methods honed on one-exposure to one-outcome paradigm, and the natural tendency to reduce a complex question to a simple answer. In the last decade multiple authors have aptly pointed out the limits to this approach, both conceptually and statistically, as people do not eat nutrients in isolation (Jacobs and Tapsell, 2007; Hu, 2002). There are further methodological points to consider, related to the advantages of studying dietary patterns rather than individual nutrients. The high correlation between many different nutrients makes it difficult, if not impossible, to draw clear nutrient-specific causal inferences (Willett, 1998). Furthermore, the effects of a single nutrient may be too small to detect in the context of an overall pattern. The translation of research on nutrients has also proven difficult since the majority of people are not capable of accurately assessing daily intake (Mozaffarian and Ludwig, 2010).

On the other hand, dietary patterns incorporate the natural collinearity observed in dietary intake, and the patterns for populations are characterized by this component of eating behavior (Hu, 2002). Moreover, examining overall dietary patterns does not fall into a pharmaceutical/reductionist approach. This is an important point to consider, given that even with the vast knowledge of nutrition, comprehensive knowledge of nutritional biochemistry in humans is incomplete (Jacobs and Tapsell, 2007). Then, again, the combination of the complexity of eating behaviors and the methods for assessment would suggest that dietary pattern information is also incomplete. Overall, conceptually and methodologically, there is a strong rationale for emphasizing dietary patterns research in relation to type 2 diabetes.

Interpreting dietary patterns and theoretical model

Central to dietary patterns research is the concept of *food synergy*, a perspective that more information can be obtained by examining foods, and the dietary patterns they make up, rather than single food or nutrient components (Jacobs and Steffen, 2003). The consideration of food synergy stems, as previously noted, form the complexity of eating as a behavior and the biological processes occurring throughout, with known and unknown levels of interactions throughout (Jacobs and Steffen, 2003, Jacobs et al., 2009). The aim of this perspective is to fundamentally understand the full effect of dietary intake on health. The crux of the perspective is that to gain full understanding and best translate dietary research into practice, it is desirable to bear in mind the overall dietary pattern, and what is known about the food groups in that pattern, individual foods, components of foods, down to specific micro-nutrients or phytochemicals such as those described elsewhere in this textbook (Jacobs et al., 2009; Jacobs and Tapsell, 2007; Jacobs and Steffen, 2003; McKeown and Jacobs, 2010).

Undeniably, dietary patterns serve as the anchor in interpreting nutrition-related research in this paradigm, but research on individual foods and nutrients should not be ignored, as it plays an important part in providing perspective and etiologic understanding. The dietary patterns/food synergy perspective may be especially germane to type 2 diabetes since this disease is not thought of as a simple excess or deficiency disease, nutrient-wise. That said, an oft-cited pillar of the viability of food synergy is the lack of effect of many isolated compounds in clinical trials (McCormick, 2010; Jacobs et al., 2009). In short, incorporating the perspective of food synergy into interpretation of the evidence based on dietary intake, we see that type 2 diabetes affords the opportunity to enhance understanding, and provides a standpoint for what really can be translated and gleaned from research. Figure 6.1 provides a theoretical model of dietary patterns intake within this perspective.

Methods for dietary patterns

This section is not meant to be exhaustive in the summary of methods employed in population-related research related to dietary patterns, but to provide a succinct overview on the topic with some key considerations to help the reader have a more complete understanding of the topic.

Two main approaches have been used to examine dietary patterns in observational epidemiological studies. One method has defined patterns a priori in index form, based upon existing evidence or knowledge on foods or nutrients. For example, different studies have derived "Mediterranean" diet scores, or "Healthy Eating Index" scores towards different chronic disease endpoints. In general, these summary indices

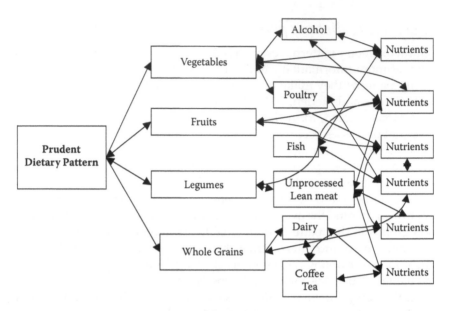

Figure 6.1 A theoretical model of a healthy dietary pattern for prevention of type 2 diabetes within the food synergy perspective. The pattern emphasizes intake of vegetables, fruits, legumes, and whole grains, with coffee and tea as beverages and, as desired, smaller amounts of dairy, fish, poultry, and unprocessed lean meat, and moderate alcohol intake. The arrows represent both synergistic and antagonistic interactions between foods, foods and nutrients, and the complexity of dietary intake.

do not reflect overall diet quality but rather selected aspects of individual nutrition (Schulze and Hoffman, 2006). One key shortcoming of using a diet quality score/index is that the quality is only relative to whatever is measured by the given index, and each index varies in terms of the dietary components that are included in the total score.

Alternatively, an empirical or a posteriori approach that relies completely on the dietary data at hand, and derives patterns based upon statistical methods is the chief source of the literature reviewed in this chapter. The method most commonly employed is *factor analysis*, a term which is used generically in much of the research in reference to either true factor analysis or *principal component analysis* (PCA). In the short history of applying these statistical data reduction techniques to nutritional research, essentially all research employing PCA or factor analysis has used food frequency questionnaire (FFQ) data, with prevalent or incident disease (e.g., type 2 diabetes) as the outcome, although it is certainly possible to examine other types of dietary data with this method.

The aim of PCA in nutritional analyses is to account for the maximal variance of dietary intake by combining the many different dietary variables into a smaller number of factors based on the intercorrelation of these variables. This approach identifies common underlying factors of food consumption. In general, PCA and factor analysis will provide similar results (Schulze and Hoffman, 2006). Patterns are typically rotated orthogonally to achieve a simple structure, uncorrelated with any other pattern derived in the analysis (Schulze and Hoffman, 2006, Norman and Streiner, 2000). Factor scores for each participant are calculated by multiplying the intake of the standardized food item by their respective factor loadings on each pattern. The loadings can be interpreted as the correlation coefficient between the food/food groups and the pattern. The scores are linear variables and represent the weighted sum of all food and beverage items assessed, and a higher score corresponds with greater conformity to the derived pattern (Norman and Streiner, 2000). These scores can be used in correlation or regression analyses.

Cluster analysis is another a posteriori/empirical method to derive dietary patterns in population-based research. However, cluster analysis has been infrequently employed in dietary patterns analysis with type 2 diabetes as an outcome. In contrast to factor analysis, cluster analysis defines exclusive clusters of individuals. These subgroups are generally homogenous and are categorized by some standardized measure relating to dietary intake (Schulze and Hoffman, 2006). The diets and related demographic and lifestyle characteristics will differ between these clusters, and this method requires further analysis and more subjective interpretation due to the different dietary profiles between clusters, as well as a lack of a natural comparison group. Due to these limitations, cluster analysis has been utilized less frequently in dietary pattern research than has factor analysis and PCA.

Reduced rank regression (RRR) is a method that has also been used in dietary pattern analysis. RRR is a hybrid between a priori and empirical analysis, and takes into account the biological pathways from diet to outcome by identifying dietary patterns associated with biomarkers or intermediates of a specific disease, then examining that diet pattern with disease occurrence. It can be interpreted as PCA applied to "responses" (Schulze and Hoffman, 2006). This method requires both intermediate and outcome data, and the number of patterns derived are limited to the number of intermediate responses. This method also provides evidence to support hypothesized pathways between dietary intake and risk of type 2 diabetes or other diseases, but should be considered complementary to empirically based dietary patterns research.

A main criticism of dietary pattern analyses is the subjective nature in the many steps that go into their development. Since the vast majority of research on dietary patterns with type 2 diabetes has used an empirical approach, what follows are major considerations and approaches researchers looking to employ this method should take into account. Certainly, formal class work, mentorship from a researcher experienced in the method, and textbooks should comprise the base of learning on this topic.

The noted aforementioned aim of dietary patterns research is to take the complexities of dietary intake as they are assessed in population studies, and distill them down to patterns defined by certain characteristics based on how people actually eat. Important considerations when beginning this type of analysis include the following:

Selection of study population. In order to minimize bias and maximize the validity of hypothesis testing, several important aspects of the study sample need to be considered. The primary points related to this issue include the sample size and number of cases that have accrued or are likely to accrue, as this will have a major influence on statistical power, as well as the level of heterogeneity of the demographics, ethnicity/race, education and income, and dietary and other lifestyle and cultural exposures. These aspects will all have a significant influence on the dietary patterns that are derived from the data, as well as on the ability to minimize biases in the estimated association between the dietary exposures and the disease outcome of interest.

A basic guideline for sample size is approximately five subjects per variable included in PCA. For example, if an FFQ has 100 items, there should be 500 participants at a minimum (Norman and Streiner, 2000). Other characteristics such as the population composition may also affect the results and need to be considered when applicable, that is, when there is potential for the pattern to be unduly influenced by factors such as, but not limited to, age, race/ethnicity, education, or smoking habits. Therefore, it is important to derive the dietary patterns after stratification by these important population characteristics that may directly or indirectly relate to, or be a marker of, dietary habits to ensure that the overall pattern structure is consistent in the population, and thus the results are generalizable across the complete study population. If the dietary patterns across these important sub-groups are shown to be consistent in loading structure, then there is no need to stratify the pattern derivation, and the analysis can be executed a final time on the entire sample to maximize statistical power.

Validity and appropriate analysis of the dietary data. On the front end, studies should exclude participants from the analysis who report extreme energy intakes that are not theoretically plausible, as well as participants who are missing significant key variables in the database. If diet was assessed with an FFQ, there should be a reasonable number of foods as well as a range of possible frequencies for the intake of the specified portions sizes for each food. Such is the essence of the "semi-quantitative FFQ." Thus, if food intake is assessed in a crude fashion, such as on a dichotomous nature (e.g., yes versus no), statistical assumptions required for PCA or factor analysis will likely be violated, and results will be of little or no value.

Food intake data: To group or not to group? This is a critical decision point where a researcher can introduce bias in the analysis and results. If the individual foods reported by the participants are subsequently grouped into broader categories ("food groups") before being analyzed by PCA or factor analysis, then the resulting dietary patterns will reflect some unknown combination of (1) how people specifically report their eating behavior, and (2) how the investigators manipulated the raw data on food intake, at least partly by subjective means. For example, whether fish and shellfish have an individual effect or contribute as part of a dietary pattern to diabetes risk is an important question. However, there are myriad ways to prepare fish and shellfish, as well as typical foods across cultures that customarily accompany them, depending on the preparation. If all fish and shellfish are grouped into one or two categories prior to PCA conflating the preparation (e.g., fried versus broiled) and correlating accompanying foods (e.g., fried potatoes versus vegetables), then the true associations between this dietary behavior and risk of type 2 diabetes may be biased. Typically this bias from misclassifying the exposure nondifferentially across subgroups in the population by those who do or do not develop diabetes, would weaken the association between exposure and outcome. This "bias towards the null" is a common bane of nutritional epidemiology.

On the other hand, the grouping of foods prior to PCA may be necessary if dietary data are based on very detailed methods collected over an extended period of time, such as multiple 24-hour recalls, or food records. A helpful example from the literature on this issue is the contradicting results observed in the Nurses' Health Study on the topic of omega-3 fatty acid intake through fish intake as reported on the food frequency questionnaire, and a "fish" dietary pattern variable. The study reported an increased risk for developing type 2 diabetes with increasing levels of omega-3 fatty acids in the diet, as well as with increasing fish intake (Kaushik et al., 2009). However, the same cohort study previously reported that higher intake of a "prudent" dietary pattern, associated with lower risk of type 2 diabetes, was characterized by higher intakes of the food groups of fruits, vegetables, legumes, fish, and poultry (Fung et al., 2004). These diverging results with respect to fish intake do not specify a particular bias, as there are many possible reasons for the differences. However, they do raise a cautionary tale for researchers. Theoretically, from a food synergy perspective, these results should not diverge. They also suggest it may be worthwhile to embrace the complexity of dietary intake and examine all foods surveyed in the analysis rather than reducing foods into groups based upon varying levels of evidence and preconceived notions of how people eat, or what "belongs" together. It is quite possible that an observed increased risk for type 2 diabetes associated with intake of omega-3 fatty acids, or the food group "fish" is confounded by fish processing and preparations that may themselves increase risk, including breading and frying of fish in oils that may contain trans fatty acids, as well as by other food items that may be eaten along with fish, such as white bread or white rice. Indeed, many fast food restaurant items include highly processed and deep-fried fish sandwiches. Although adjustments are made for as many of these confounding factors as are measured and available in the database, residual confounding—the result of unmeasured or poorly measured confounders—is a common problem in this field.

What number of factors or dietary patterns should be retained for analysis? Underlying the following interpretative decision points is that factors should be rotated orthogonally (so the patterns are uncorrelated). There are other rotational options and approaches, when implementing a different approach that can be used, one will need to be mindful of what the rotated data represent. The number of factors to retain is based on eigenvalues, examined with a "scree plot," and individual factor loadings and factorial complexity. These decisions are arbitrary within a certain framework, but do have a statistical basis. For example, all eigenvalues should be >1.0 so that they account for more variance than is generated by 1 variable (Norman and Streiner, 2000). The scree plot is used as an eye-ball test of eigenvalues plotted against the factors. The suggested method for this test is to retain those factors with the highest eigenvalues until there is a noticeable point of inflection in the curve of points on the plot. By way of example, Figure 6.2 displays a scree plot that was used in the derivation of dietary patterns using PCA on data from the Singapore Chinese Health Study (Odegaard et al., 2011). Two factors were identified that had the highest eigenvalues and were clearly above a point of inflection, change of slope, in the eigenvalue curve. The findings for dietary patterns and type 2 diabetes risk that evolved from this analysis will be described later.

Once the pattern or patterns have been identified based on the scree plot, the next step is to interrogate the food composition of the patterns being considered for retention in the analysis. Review of the loading structure, the next step in the process, involves examining the correlation of individual foods/dishes with the overall pattern score that is comprised of those foods. If multiple foods are loading strongly (e.g., r > 0.20) on different

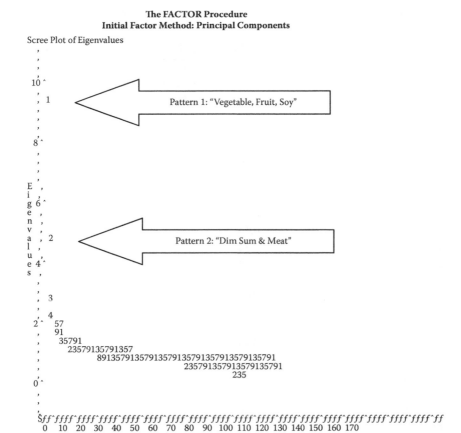

The FACTOR Procedure
Initial Factor Method: Principal Components

Figure 6.2 Example of a scree plot from principal components analysis of dietary data from The Singapore Chinese Health Study.

patterns, they may be considered "factorially complex," making it difficult to interpret the role of the food and thus the overall dietary patterns in relation to the outcome. There is no prescribed method for dealing with factorial complexity in nutritional epidemiology; other fields employing this method will sometimes use different types of rotation to confirm complexity, while also being mindful of what the data from different rotational approaches represents. That said, there is nothing violated with factorial complexity from a mathematical standpoint; rather, it is a consideration for interpretative simplicity. Overall, cautious interpretation should be emphasized If this is observed in a study, especially if there are large age ranges or heterogeneous subpopulations of race/ethnicity, since this may represent underlying different eating habits. An example of the loading structure for two dietary patterns derived in the Singapore Chinese Health Study (Odegaard et al., 2011) is shown in Table 6.1.

Table 6.1 Factor Loadings for Foods with Vegetable, Fruit, and Soy Rich-Dietary Pattern in Singapore Chinese Health Study (VFS)

Food item	Food type	Loading	Food item	Food type	Loading
Cauliflower	V	0.54	Fried vegetarian beehoon	St, V	0.20
Broccoli	V	0.49	Soy bean drink	S	0.20
Carrots	V	0.49			
Green beans/peas	V	0.48			
Other plain tofu	S	0.46			
Yin choi, po choi	V	0.43			
Corn	V	0.43			
Tung goo	O, Pr	0.43			
Tomatoes	V	0.42			
Gum jum, dried fungus	O, Pr	0.42			
White potatoes	V, St	0.41			
Head lettuce, Chinese lettuce	V	0.41			
Kai lan	V	0.40			
Other tau kwa	S	0.40			
Tou gay, tai tau nga	V	0.40			
Pak choy, siew pak choy	V	0.40			
Choi sum	V	0.40			
Fu kua, mo qua	V	0.38			
Head cabbage, wong nga pak	V	0.38			
Watercress	V	0.37			
Foojook vegetarian meats	S	0.37			
Celery	V	0.37			
Kai choi	V	0.35			
Cucumber	V	0.34			
Apples	F	0.34			
Other tau pok	S	0.32			
Yong tau foo	S	0.31			
Papaya	F	0.31			
Pears	F	0.31			

Table 6.1 Factor Loadings for Foods with Vegetable, Fruit, and Soy Rich-Dietary Pattern in Singapore Chinese Health Study (VFS) (continued)

Food item	Food type	Loading	Food item	Food type	Loading
Other dark green leaves	V	0.31			
Canned baked beans	L	0.30			
Honeydew	F	0.30			
Gee choi	V	0.29			
Bananas	F	0.29			
Watermelon	F	0.28			
Grapes	F	0.28			
Boiled/steamed fish	Fi	0.27			
Fish ball/cake	Fi	0.27			
Oranges	F	0.27			
Ung choi	V	0.26			
Onions	V	0.26			
Chinese chives	V, O	0.26			
Tofu far	S	0.25			
Pan-/stir-fried chicken	P	0.25			
Ikan bilis	Pr, Fi	0.22			

Note: Definitions of abbreviations: B—beverage; C—condiment; Da—dairy; DS—dim sum/snack dish; F—fruit; Fi—fish/shellfish/seafood; L—legumes; M—meat; O—other; P—poultry; Pr—preserved; S—soy food; St—high starch item (e.g., noodle dish, rice dish); Sw—sweet; WG—whole grain.

* Factor loads correspond to Pearson correlation coefficients between the food and the respective dietary pattern.

Epidemologic Studies of dietary patterns and type 2 diabetes risk

Over the last decade a diverse array of studies has examined the question of overall dietary patterns with risk of developing type 2 diabetes. Discussion of the following literature focuses on those studies that have included empirically derived dietary patterns. The salient features of the individual studies and a summary of their findings can be found in Table 6.2.

The first prospective cohort study to report on overall dietary patterns and risk for incident type 2 diabetes was The Health Professionals Follow-Up Study (van Dam et al., 2002). This study included 42,504 male health professionals aged 40–75 years who were free of major chronic

Table 6.2 Factor Loadings for Foods with Dim-Sum and Meat-Rich Dietary Pattern in Singapore Chinese Health Study (DSM)

Food item	Food type	Loading	Food item	Food type	Loading
Siew mai	DS, M	0.44	Fresh Chilis	C	0.21
Other steamed snack	DS, M	0.42	Chee cheong fun	DS,M	0.21
Gravy noodle	St, M	0.42	Watermelon	F	0.21
Chicken rice	St, P	0.41	Other pork	M	0.20
Otar otar	DS	0.39	Ung choi	V	0.20
Chicken, mutton curry	M	0.39	Salted roots	Pr, V	0.20
Steamed meat bao	DS, M	0.38	Balachan	C	0.20
Glutinous rice dumpling	St, M	0.38	Other dried seafood	Fi, Pr	0.20
Pork satay	M	0.37	Flavored rice porridge	St	0.20
Roasted duck or goose	P	0.36	Deep-fried fish	Fi	0.20
Popiah	DS, M	0.36	Baked buns w/meat	St, M	0.20
Other pig organs (intestine)	M	0.35	Hot dogs	M, Pr	0.20
Ngor hiang	DS, M	0.35			
Preserved eggs	O, Pr	0.35			
Roti prata	St	0.35			
Chinese rojak	DS, V	0.35			
Puffs, curry, or bean	DS, V	0.34			
Coconut rice	St	0.34			
Deep-fried chicken	P	0.34			
Other flavored rice	St, M	0.34			
Dry noodle dish	St, M	0.34			
Chicken satay	P	0.33			
Curry rice	St	0.33			
Coconut desserts	DS, Sw	0.32			
Belly pork	M	0.32			
Deep-fried snacks	DS	0.32			

Table 6.2 Factor Loadings for Foods with Dim-Sum and Meat-Rich Dietary Pattern in Singapore Chinese Health Study (DSM) (continued)

Food item	Food type	Loading	Food item	Food type	Loading
Other fried noodle	St, M, Fi	0.31			
Lup chong	M	0.31			
Luncheon meat	M	0.30			
Squid	Fi	0.29			
Soft drinks	B, Sw	0.29			
Fried rice	St	0.28			
Canned sardine	Fi	0.28			
Sweet kuey	DS, Sw	0.28			
Pork liver	M	0.27			
Salted fish	Fi, Pr	0.26			
Shrimp	Fi	0.26			
Eggs	O	0.26			
French fries	St, O	0.25			
Steamed sweet bao	DS, Sw	0.25			
Red/green bean soups	DS	0.25			
Ice cream/ frozen yogurt	Da, Sw	0.25			
Pineapple	F	0.22			
Western cakes	DS, Sw	0.22			
Hamburgers	M	0.22			

Note: Definitions of abbreviations: B—beverage; C—condiment; Da—dairy; DS—dim sum/snack dish; F—fruit; Fi—fish/shellfish/seafood; L—legumes; M—meat; O—other; P—poultry; Pr—preserved; S—soy food; St—high starch item (e.g., noodle dish, rice dish); Sw—sweet; WG—whole grain.

Factor loads correspond to Pearson correlation coefficients between the food and the respective dietary pattern.

disease at baseline in 1986, and did not report extreme energy intakes. This is one of the rare studies that assessed dietary intake multiple times through a 131-item FFQ, whereas most cohort studies have only one baseline dietary assessment. Foods were grouped from the FFQ into 37 predefined groups similar in nutrient profile and culinary use. Factor analysis was employed to derive the dietary patterns. Diabetes was self-reported and validated, and participants were followed through 1998. Two major dietary patterns were derived. One was labeled a "prudent" pattern and was characterized by high consumption of vegetables, fruits, fish, poultry, and whole grains, and the other was termed "western" and characterized by high consumption of red meat, processed meat, high-fat dairy products, French fries, refined grains, and sweetened foods. The prudent pattern was suggestively associated with a reduced risk of developing type 2 diabetes. The western pattern was associated with a strong increased risk of type 2 diabetes, and these results were stronger in older men, those with a family history of type 2 diabetes, low physical activity and higher body mass index. This study was soundly executed with no major limitations, other than the potential problems that could arise in interpretation due to the grouping of foods into groups prior to conducting PCA, as discussed earlier. However, it is worth considering the possible implications of the investigators' decision to include alcohol intake as a covariate in the model, when it was also included as a food group in the dietary patterns analysis. It is unclear if this approach would have any substantial effect on the results. From a theoretical perspective the approach may misclassify the contribution of alcohol intake to the dietary pattern.

The Nurses' Health Study has also examined dietary patterns with risk of incident type 2 diabetes (Fung et al., 2004). The study included 69,554 women free of major chronic disease aged 38–63 in 1984 who did not report extreme dietary intake. Diet was assessed multiple times through a 116 item FFQ and participants were followed through 1998. Diabetes was self-reported and validated. Foods were grouped and factor analysis was the analytic approach used to derive dietary patterns. A prudent and western pattern, both highly alike the patterns from the Health Profession Study were derived. As well, similar analytic approaches, and results were observed. The prudent pattern had a moderate, suggestive inverse association with risk of type 2 diabetes, whereas there was a strong positive association between the western pattern and diabetes risk. Heavier women with a family history of diabetes were observed to have a stronger risk with greater adherence to a western dietary pattern. Overall, this study mirrors the Health Professionals Study in being soundly conducted, and having the same minor potential limitations.

A study of 4,304 Finnish men and women aged 40–69 and free of diabetes in 1967–72 were followed for 23 years, with PCA-derived dietary patterns modeled in association with incident diabetes risk (Montonen et al., 2005). Habitual dietary intake was assessed in a dietary history interview of over 100 food items, which where were then combined into groups. Diabetes was identified from a nationwide registry. Two dietary patterns were derived: a "prudent" pattern characterized by high intakes of vegetables, fruits, and poultry, and a "conservative" pattern characterized by high intake of butter, potatoes, whole milk, rye, other grains, and processed meat. The prudent pattern was inversely associated with risk of diabetes, and the conservative pattern positively associated with diabetes risk. A few methodological points related to this study include the observation that a number of the food groups were factorially complex, and the diabetes cases were only those who received drug reimbursements, which suggests they were likely the more severe cases. Overall, this study was well executed but plausible reasons for the factorial complexity may stem from the grouping of foods prior to PCA, or less heterogeneity in the overall diet.

The Melbourne Collaborative Cohort study has also published a study on dietary patterns and type 2 diabetes risk (Hodge et al., 2007). This study included 31,641 men and women aged 27–75 (99% were 40–69) with significant subpopulations of migrants from Italy and Greece (to go along with native Australians and United Kingdom citizens) enrolled from 1990 to 1994 and followed for 4 years. Participants were all free of major chronic disease and did not report extreme dietary intake. Dietary assessment was conducted with a 121-item FFQ developed specifically for this cohort. Diabetes was self-reported and used a variety of methods to ascertain status. Principal component analysis was used to derive dietary patterns and was performed on all 121 individual items, which is the strength of this analysis if using the rationale noted above. Four patterns were derived, with a pattern characterized by higher intakes of processed grains, red and processed meats, and fried foods being positively associated with diabetes risk, and a pattern characterized by whole grains, dairy, poultry, steamed fish, vegetables, and fruits displaying a suggestive inverse association. The patterns were associated with the different ethnic groups in the study, and the adjustment of both body mass index and waist/hip ratio in the same model were two methodological points of concern. Such adjustment may obscure the true association between dietary intake and diabetes risk due to body composition likely being involved in the causal pathway between diet and diabetes risk. One can not attempt to tease out dietary effects that may be due to body composition versus those that may be independent of body composition unless a series of models are presented with and without adjustment for such variables as body mass index and waist/hip ratio. A final minor concern that causes some difficulty in interpreting the findings is that a number of food items loaded strongly on more than one pattern.

Investigators from the MESA study have also examined empirical dietary patterns with type 2 diabetes (Nettleton et al., 2008). This multicenter study in the United States included 5,011 men and women of Caucasian, African-American, Hispanic, and Chinese ethnicity aged 45–84 at baseline in 2000–2002 and followed through 2007. Usual dietary intake was assessed with a 120-item FFQ, with 47 food groups defined by the investigators prior to PCA. The diabetes case definition comprised self-report, diabetic fasting glucose at the exam, or use of medication. Four dietary patterns were derived. A beans, tomatoes, and refined grains pattern was suggestively associated in quartiles of score with greater risk of diabetes, and associated with an increased risk per standard deviation increase in the score. A whole grains and fruit pattern was inversely associated with diabetes risk. A concern with the results is the potential influence of race/ethnicity differentially affecting the patterns and risk for diabetes, given the propensity of persons of African-American, Hispanic, and Asian ancestry to be at higher risk for diabetes relative to Caucasians and other groups. There was no evidence of formal statistical effect modification by race/ethnicity, although the results were suggestive of such effect modification by race/ethnicity given the sample size and distribution of the population. There was also evidence of factorial complexity in the loading of food groups on the different factors, which again may be an artifact of investigator-derived food groups prior to carrying out PCA. Overall, the study was soundly executed, and the aforementioned considerations and limitations may have been unavoidable given the population and data at hand.

Few nonwestern population-based studies have reported on the association between dietary patterns and type 2 diabetes. The first was the Shanghai Women's Health Study, which included 64,191 Chinese women aged 40–70, free of major chronic disease without extreme reports of energy intake (Villegas et al., 2010). A 77-item FFQ, developed and validated in the population assessed usual dietary intake. Eleven food groups were created and included in cluster analysis. Three clusters or patterns were derived. Type 2 diabetes was self-reported. Compared to a cluster with greater rice, less meat and seafood, fruit, vegetable, dairy, and snack and dessert intake, a cluster with greater fruit and vegetables, dairy, meat, and seafood, and less soy and rice was associated with a decreased risk. Because of the approach (cluster analysis), it is difficult to differentiate whether the results are due to diet or due to other characteristics related to dietary habits, that is, residual confounding. Recall that, unlike PCA, cluster analysis results in distinct subgroups of the population based on heterogeneity between individuals in eating habits.

The Singapore Chinese Health Study also examined empirical dietary patterns with risk of type 2 diabetes in 43,176 Chinese men and women, aged 45–74 at baseline in 1993–98, free of major chronic disease, and followed up through 2004 (Odegaard et al., 2011). A 165-item FFQ specifically designed for and validated in the study population assessed usual dietary intake. The PCA of all 165 foods, dishes, and beverages was used to derive a vegetable–fruit–soy (VFS)–rich pattern characterized by high levels of vegetables, fruit, soy foods, and seafood, and a dim sum- and meat-rich (DSM) pattern characterized by high levels of dim sum, meat and processed meat, fried foods, and sweetened foods and beverages. The results of the associations with diabetes incidence were significantly modified by smoking status, with no association observed in ever smokers (27.4% of the sample) for either dietary pattern. In nonsmokers (72.6% of the sample), a strong inverse association was observed between the VFS pattern and type 2 diabetes risk, whereas a strong positive association was observed between the DSM pattern and diabetes risk.

In the Multiethnic Cohort Study based in Hawaii, 75,512 Japanese-Americans, Native Hawaiians, and Caucasians enrolled in a study of diet and cancer (Erber et al., 2010). Participants were aged 45–75, free of major chronic disease, and without extreme reported dietary intake. Diabetes was ascertained by questionnaires, and linkage was conducted with major health plans. The FFQ was developed and validated in the population but was of unreported length. Food groups were created, and then PCA was used to derive the dietary patterns. Three different patterns were derived, and results were examined by ethnic group and sex. Overall, a fat and meat pattern characterized by organ meats, processed meats, discretionary fat, white potatoes, and processed grains was associated with an increased risk of diabetes. A pattern rich in vegetables and fruits was generally associated with an inverse association. A third pattern, rich in fruits and dairy was suggestively associated with a lower risk of diabetes. None of the factors showed any association in Native Hawaiians, and there was evidence of trends across the ethnic groups. The factors were derived in a simplified approach, where food groups not loading over a prespecified, arbitrary level were excluded from the final pattern, and thus did not contribute to the pattern score. Still, the patterns were factorially complex, as was noted in several of the other studies described. Another methodological issue was the exclusion of nearly 8,700 participants of undefined ethnicity who were eligible for the study.

The final study identified was of modest size and is thus not included in Table 6.2 due to limited statistical power. This study included 690 Hong Kong Chinese men and women aged 25–74 (Yu et al., 2011). Diet was assessed with a 266-item FFQ, and diabetes was assessed by glucose measurement. PCA was used to derive dietary patterns. Despite the lack of power, the results had face validity as a dietary pattern characterized by vegetables, fruit, and fish was suggestively associated with reduced risk of type 2 diabetes, and a pattern characterized by meat and dairy products was suggestively associated with an increased risk.

Complementary to the empirical dietary patterns research are four studies that approached this question using reduced rank regression (McNaughton et al., 2008; Schulze et al., 2005; Liese et al., 2009; Heidemann et al., 2005). All have derived patterns explaining the greatest variation in biomarkers for inflammation, insulin resistance, glycemia, or lipids. All observed inverse or positive associations with diabetes risk in the nested case control studies, but with generally less precision than the larger empirical based dietary pattern studies. The patterns aligned with the aforementioned summarized studies in content. The Nurses' Health Study appears to be the only study to examine this question using empirically-derived patterns as well as reduced rank regression. The results derived with reduced rank regression were consistent with the Western dietary pattern derived using factor analysis (Fung et al., 2004; Schulze et al., 2005). These results support the complementary role of reduced rank regression, and also pleiotropic role of an overall dietary pattern, as they are clearly related across multiple pathways. Thus, reduced rank regression has shown to be an important confirmatory research tool. Continued research employing reduced rank regression will certainly contribute to understanding known and novel diet–diabetes pathways.

Conclusion

Appreciation of, and research on, overall dietary patterns in health, and specifically type 2 diabetes has picked up steam over the last decade. There are a number of important considerations that go along with this research that are conceptual and methodological. Based on data from the study of dietary patterns in prospective cohort studies, it can be said with confidence that recommending a pattern emphasizing vegetables, fruits, legumes, whole grains, nuts, and including (not in excess) dairy, varieties of seafood, unprocessed poultry, red meat and oils from fruits/nuts/seeds (e.g., olive, canola) is beneficial; whereby a dietary pattern emphasizing sweetened foods and beverages, processed grains, cured meats, fatty meats, and deep fried foods increases risk. These dietary pattern characteristics were consistent across very different populations who have different geographical, political, demographic, socio–economic, and ethnic/racial characteristics, and thus different propensities for diabetes. A take-home public health and prevention of diabetes message on the topic would emphasize a healthy overall dietary pattern within an appropriate cultural context. Such an approach, if focused on upstream policies that are bold yet realistic, is quite likely to have a trickle-down impact on the risk factors for type 2 diabetes, such as obesity and insulin resistance, and thus a down-stream public health impact on risk for type 2 diabetes, as well as cardiovascular disease and possibly certain cancers. Continued research will hone this topic, and address important questions such as whether a "healthy" or "unhealthy" dietary pattern modifies genetic susceptibility towards type 2 diabetes. Despite their nascent status in the world of nutritional research, dietary patterns hold much hope to serve as the basis for dietary recommendations for prevention of type 2 diabetes.

References

Erber, E., Hopping, B. N, Grandinetti, A., Park, S. Y., Kolonel, L. N., and Maskarinec, G. 2010. Dietary patterns and risk for diabetes: The multiethnic cohort. *Diabetes Care*, 33, 532–8.

Fung, T., Schulze, M., Manson, J. E., Willett, W. C., and Hu, F. B. 2004. Dietary patterns, meat intake, and the risk of type 2 diabetes in women. *Arch Intern Med,* 164, 2235–40.

Heidemann, C., Hoffmann, K., Spranger, J., Klipstein-Grobusch, K., Möhlig, M., Pfeiffer, A. F., and Boeing, H. 2005. A dietary pattern protective against type 2 diabetes in the European Prospective Investigation into Cancer and Nutrition (EPIC)—Potsdam Study cohort. *Diabetologia,* 48, 1126–34.

Hodge, A. M., English, D. R., O'Dea, K., and Giles, G. G. 2007. Dietary patterns and diabetes incidence in the Melbourne collaborative cohort study. *Am J Epidemiol,* 165, 603–610.

Hu, F. B. 2002. Dietary pattern analysis: A new direction in nutritional epidemiology. *Curr Opin Lipidol,* 13, 3–9.

Jacobs, D. R., Jr., and Steffen, L. M. 2003. Nutrients, foods, and dietary patterns as exposures in research: A framework for food synergy. *Am J Clin Nutr,* 78, 508S–513S.

Jacobs, D. R., Jr., Gross, M. D., and Tapsell, L. C. 2009. Food synergy: An operational concept for understanding nutrition. *Am J Clin Nutr,* 89 (suppl.), 1s–6s.

Jacobs, D. R., Jr., and Tapsell, L. C. 2007. Food, not nutrients, is the fundamental unit in nutrition. *Nutr Rev,* 65, 439–50.

Kaushik, M., Mozaffarian, D., Spiegelman, D., Manson, J. E., Willett, W. C., and Hu, F. B. 2009. Long-chain omega-3 fatty acids, fish intake, and the risk of type 2 diabetes mellitus. *Am J Clin Nutr,* 90, 613–20.

Liese, A. D., Weis, K. E., Schulz, M., and Tooze, J. A. 2009. Food intake patterns associated with incident type 2 diabetes: The Insulin Resistance Atherosclerosis Study. *Diabetes Care,* 32, 263–8.

McCormick, D. B. 2010. Vitamin/mineral supplements: Of questionable benefit for the general population. *Nutr Rev,* 68, 207–13.

McKeown, N. M., and Jacobs, D. R. 2010. In defence of phytochemical-rich dietary patterns. *Br J Nutr,* 104, 1–3.

McNaughton, S. A., Mishra, G. D., and Brunner, E. J. 2008. Dietary patterns, insulin resistance, and incidence of type 2 diabetes in the Whitehall II study. *Diabetes Care,* 31, 1343–48.

Montonen, J., Knekt, P., Härkänen, T., Järvinen, R., Heliövaara, M., Aromaa, A., and Reunanen, A. 2005. Dietary patterns and the incidence of type 2 diabetes. *Am J Epidemiol,* 161, 219–27.

Mozaffarian, D., and Ludwig, D. S. 2010. Dietary guidelines in the 21st century—a time for food. *JAMA,* 304, 1–2.

Nestle, M. 2002. *Food Politics: How the Food Industry Influences Nutrition and Health.* Berkeley, University of California Press.

Nettleton, J. A., Steffen, L. M., Ni, H., Liu, K., and Jacobs, J. R., Dr. 2008. Dietary patterns and risk of incident type 2 diabetes in the multi-ethnic study of atherosclerosis (MESA). *Diabetes Care,* 31, 1777–82.

Norman, G. R., and Streiner, D. L. 2000. *Biostatistics. The Bare Essentials.* Hamilton, Ontario, BC Decker.

Odegaard, A. O., Koh, W. P., Butler, L. M., Duval, S., Gross, M. D., Yu, M. C., Yuan, J. M., Pereira, M. A. 2011. Dietary patterns and incident type 2 diabetes in Chinese men and women: The Singapore Chinese Health Study. *Diabetes Care,* 34, 880–85.

Schulze, M. B., Hoffman, K, Manson, J. E., Willett, W. C., Meigs, J. B., Weikert, C., Heidemann, C., Colditz, G. A., and Hu, F. B. 2005. Dietary pattern, inflammation, and incidence of type 2 diabetes in women. *Am J Clin.*

Schulze, M. B., and Hoffman, K. 2006. Methodological approaches to study dietary patterns in relation to risk of coronary heart disease and stroke. *Br J Nutr*, 95, 860–69.

Van Dam, R. M., Rimm, E. B., Willett, W. C., Stampfer, M. J., and Hu, F. B. 2002. Dietary patterns and risk for type 2 diabetes mellitus in U.S. men. *Ann Intern Med*, 136, 201–9.

Villegas, R., Yang G., Gao, Y. T., Cai, H., Li, H., Zheng, W., and SHU, X. O. 2010. Dietary patterns are associated with lower incidence of type 2 diabetes in middle-aged women: The Shanghai Women's Health Study. *Int J Epidem*, 39, 889–99.

Willett, W. C. 1998. *Nutritional Epidemiology*. New York, Oxford University Press.

Yu, R., Woo, J., Chan, R., Sham, A., Ho, S., Tso, A., Cheung, B., Lam, T. H., and Lam, K. 2011. Relationship between dietary intake and the development of type 2 diabetes in a Chinese population: The Hong Kong Dietary Survey. *Public Health Nutr*, 5, 1–9.

chapter seven

Special topics:
Artificially sweetened beverages and coffee

Mark A. Pereira, PhD

Noel T. Mueller, MPH

Andrew O. Odegaard, PhD
University of Minnesota

Contents

A description of the purported mechanisms and the scientific evidence on the link between sugar-sweetened beverages (SSB) and risk of type 2 diabetes was covered in Chapter 2, as SSB are one of the leading contributors to intake of simple sugars in the United States and many other developed countries. This chapter focuses on two other types of popular beverages for which relevant and recent scientific evidence has accumulated in the area of diabetes etiology and risk. These beverages, artificially sweetened beverages (ASB) and coffee, are not covered elsewhere in this book because they typically contain little or no macronutrients or energy other than what may be added to them by the consumer.

Artificially sweetened beverages

ASB are marketed and used as a replacement for SSB, and are suggested through advertisements to be helpful for weight loss and diabetes prevention or control. The sweeteners used in ASB are potent—at least 100 times the sweetness of sucrose. Six artificial sweeteners have been deemed safe for human consumption by the U.S. Food and Drug Administration (FDA), including acesulfame potassium, aspartame, saccharin, sucralose, neotame, and stevia (Rebaudioside A or rebiana).

Among both youth and adults, those who consume more ASB tend to have higher relative body weight, and are more likely to be dieting to lose weight (Bleich, Wang et al. 2009; Vanselow, Pereira et al. 2009; de Koning, Malik et al. 2011; Mozaffarian, Hao et al. 2011). Intake of ASB increases with age (Popkin 2010) and is more common in diabetics versus nondiabetics (Mackenzie et al. 2006). Consistent with their reported attempts at weight loss, those who with higher ASB intake tend to report healthier dietary habits (Lutsey, Steffen et al. 2008; Vanselow, Pereira et al. 2009; de Koning, Malik et al. 2011). Cross-sectional studies are therefore of little use in studying this topic because of the likely biases that cannot be addressed due to the lack of temporality in the study design.

Whether coincidental or causal with respect to the increasing rates of obesity and diabetes, intake of beverages has changed drastically over the past several decades. Increases in SSB such as soft drinks, colas, other sweetened carbonated beverages, and fruit drinks with added sugar have steadily increased in frequency and portion sizes, especially among youth, where a parallel decline in cow's milk has occurred (Harnack, Stang et al. 1999; Yen and Lin 2002; French, Lin et al. 2003). However, with respect to ASB, the trends are less clear, and this may be due to having less population-based data on ASB as a specific exposure. Some evidence suggests there has been a steady increase in consumption of ASB over the last several decades (Mattes and Popkin 2009; Popkin 2010), whereas other national surveys suggest stability, and perhaps decline, in the prevalence in ASB intake since the early 1990s (Mattes and Popkin 2009).

Potential mechanisms

It has been hypothesized that ASB may increase weight gain and diabetes risk through a dysregulation of appetite control due to the mismatch between the intense taste of sweetness during consumption and the lack of energy that is consumed. As such, ASB intake could lead to overcompensation of solid foods, alterations of taste sensations or preferences, blunting of a cephalic phase response, and *Pavlovian conditioning* with respect to hedonics, pleasures, or rewards (Mattes and Popkin 2009; Swithers et al. 2010). Short-term mechanistic trials in animals and humans have provided some etiological insights as a basis for further study of the possible effects of ASB on appetite dysregulation and weight-gain (Ludwig 2009; Mattes and Popkin 2009). Rodent models have provided some evidence in support of these (Swithers et al. 2010). However, as discussed below, the evidence in humans is more sparse and less consistent (Renwick and Molinary 2010; Tordoff and Alleva 1990; Raben 2002; Mattes and Popkin 2009).

Specific to diabetes etiology is the potential effect of ASB on the gut incretin hormones, specifically glucagon-like peptide-1 (GLP-1) and gastric inhibitory polypeptide (GIP). In addition to their oral location, sweet taste receptors are also found in the lining of the gut (Nelson et al. 2001), and both nutritive (sugar) and nonnutritive (used in ASB) sweeteners may stimulate these receptors, present on the GLP-1 secreting L-cells, and thus potential to influence GLP-1 secretion and glycemic dynamics (Jang et al. 2007; Brown et al. 2009). The evidence supporting this pathway appears to be limited to animals, as human studies have not been able to replicate stimulation of incretins via intra-gastric or oral routes (Ma et al. 2009). Thus, in humans orally ingested or intra-gastrically infused artificial sweeteners do not appear to stimulate incretins or other gut hormones (Ford et al. 2011; Steinert et al. 2011). This lack of stimulation of incretins by artificial sweeteners either orally or via the gut may be due to the lack of concurrent energy intake in these studies. On the other hand, the concept of using nonnutritive sweetener preloads to stimulate greater GLP-1 and GIP secretion and thus potentially impact postprandial glycemic excursions is a developing concept that holds promise for mechanistic insight with respect to diabetes etiology.

One study tested the effect of sweet preloads ingested before consumption of a standard carbohydrate-based meal to examine the effects on incretin and accompanying insulin secretion, gastric emptying, and postprandial glycemic excursion in healthy adults. The preload, *sucralose*, did not increase secretion of GLP-1 and thus resulted in lower levels of insulin secretion and quicker gastric emptying relative to glucose and other sweet substrates (Wu et al. 2012). In another study, a full serving of a commercial ASB consumed as a preload by healthy young adults resulted in significantly enhanced GLP-1 secretion, and suggested higher insulin levels relative to water (Brown et al. 2009). However, the glucose excursions were not different. Future studies capturing any effects on the incretin response and related glucose/insulin excursion from a preload of ASB prior to glucose/food consumption would provide insight into an intriguing and developing area of study. The above described pathways provide plausible hypotheses for a possible role for ASB in modulating risk for type 2 diabetes. However, these are very difficult areas to study well in human experiments.

Prospective cohort studies of ASB and body weight

Five prospective cohort studies have reported on ASB intake and body weight change or obesity risk in youth (Ludwig et al. 2001; Berkey et al. 2004; Blum, Jacobsen et al. 2005; Striegel-Moore, Thompson et al. 2006; Vanselow, Pereira et al. 2009). The first study published on this topic, by Ludwig et al. (2001), estimated the odds of becoming obese over 19 months was reduced by 56% (OR = 0.44, p = .03) for each serving per day increase in ASB. The opposite finding was observed in the cohort study by Blum et al. (Blum, Jacobsen et al. 2005) in which ASB was the only beverage associated positively with BMI at the 2-year follow-up assessment in their cohort of youth. It is quite possible, due to the observation described earlier of those trying to lose weight being more likely to consume ASB than those not attempting weight loss (Stice, Cameron et al. 1999; Field, Austin et al. 2003; Stice, Presnell et al. 2005; Neumark-Sztainer, Wall et al. 2006), that a positive association between ASB intake and weight gain may be explained by bias due to *reverse causality*, or bias resulting from the outcome, in this case weight gain or obesity risk, having an effect on the exposure (i.e., ASB consumption). Indeed, Vanselow and colleagues (Vanselow, Pereira et al. 2009) observed a positive association between ASB intake and weight-gain over 5 years in the Project EAT cohort study of Minneapolis/St. Paul (Minnesota) school children, only to demonstrate that this association was weakened and no longer statistically significant after adjusting for dieting behaviors and weight loss concerns (Vanselow, Pereira et al. 2009). It seems that ASB may be positively associated with obesity risk in some studies only because those trying to control their weight use ASB as one of their strategies, and the overall success rate in achieving weight loss among the overweight and obese is typically poor.

Among the few cohort studies on this topic in adults, the results are also quite mixed (Choi et al. 2008; Fowler, Williams et al. 2008; Nettleton, Lutsey et al. 2009; Mozaffarian, Hao et al. 2011). The study by Nettleton et al. did not consider reverse causality by dieting behavior (Nettleton, Lutsey et al. 2009). Data from the San Antonio Heart Study supported graded, positive associations between NSB and weight gain or obesity among adults, and this association appeared to be consistent for those who were or were not dieting at baseline (Fowler, Williams et al. 2008). However, this study has a number of important limitations, including lack of repeated assessments of diet intake or dieting behavior and lack of adjustment for other dietary beverages or dietary components (Fowler,

Williams et al. 2008). Thus, questions still remain about confounding, reverse causality, and other possible biases.

In the Nurses Health Study II, 51,603 female adults were analyzed for weight change from 1991 to 1999, with weight, heights, and diabetes being self-reported, and diet measured by an extensive validated food frequency questionnaire over time (Schulze et al. 2004). Weight gain in participants who increased their ASB consumption from one drink or less per week in 1991 to one drink or more per day in 1995 (1.59 kg) was significantly lower compared with women who decreased their diet soft drink consumption from one drink or more per day in 1991 to one drink or less per week in 1995 (4.25 kg) (*P*<.001). Similar results were observed in a pooled analysis of 120,877 adult women and men from the Nurses Health Study I and II, and the Health Professionals Follow-Up Study (Mozaffarian, Hao et al. 2011). Thus, although the studies in youth and adults are not entirely consistent, those of highest quality and that used repeated measures of diet and body weight, and took into account reverse causality, suggest an inverse (protective) association between ASB and body weight change or obesity risk.

Randomized controlled trials of ASB and body weight

At least three randomized trials of ASB and body weight have been performed in youth (James, Thomas et al. 2004; Ebbeling, Feldman et al. 2006; Sichieri, Paula Trotte et al. 2009). Two of these trials were group-randomized school-based educational interventions for one year (James, Thomas et al. 2004; Sichieri, Paula Trotte et al. 2009), while the other was a home-based 6-month intervention that provided water and ASB to normal weight and overweight children who were recruited based on their relatively high intake of SSB at baseline (Ebbeling, Feldman et al. 2006). All three studies noted no overall effect on change in body mass. Interestingly, the trials by Sichieri et al. (2009) and by Ebbeling et al. (James, Thomas et al. 2004) both observed an intervention effect for the subset who were overweight or obese, providing a suggestion for a plausible interaction between the intervention and susceptibility to weight gain among certain individuals.

There have been four randomized controlled trials comparing effects of ASB and SSB consumption on body weight in adults (Tordoff and Alleva 1990; DiMeglio and Mattes 2000; Raben, Vasilaras et al. 2002; Maersk, Belza et al. 2012; Tate, Turner-McGrievy et al. 2012). The studies were relatively small and short term, with the exception of the recent trial by Tate et al. (Tate, Turner-McGrievy et al. 2012), which included 318 adults for 6 months. Two of the studies observed a significant effect on body weight (Tordoff and Alleva 1990; Raben, Vasilaras et al. 2002), favoring modestly higher weight-gain for the SSB group relative to the active intervention group of replacing SSB with ASB, milk, or water.

ASB consumption and risk for T2D in epidemiologic cohort studies

Several studies in adults have examined the association between ASB and risk of chronic disease and risk factors, including incidence of type 2 diabetes or the development of risk factors for diabetes and cardiovascular disease. Among 6,154 adult men and women of the Framingham Heart Study, both SSB and ASB appeared to increase the risk of metabolic syndrome, the potential for clustering of risk factors for T2D and cardiovascular disease, and development by ~50%, a finding that was statistically significant for ASB but not for SSB (Dhingra, Sullivan et al. 2007). Findings were similar in the ARIC Study, with a strong association between ASB and metabolic syndrome risk than for SSB and metabolic syndrome risk (Lutsey, Steffen et al. 2008). However, while findings from the Multi-Ethnic Study of Atherosclerosis in 5,011 adults of White, African American, Hispanic, and Chinese descent appeared to be consistent for ASB and metabolic syndrome association, closer examination of the individual components of the metabolic syndrome revealed some inconsistencies in the data (Nettleton, Lutsey et al. 2009). While ASB were associated with central obesity and high blood glucose, they were not associated with hypertension, hypertriglyceridemia, or low HDL cholesterol concentrations, suggesting that there is a possible association between ASB and obesity and diabetes risk, but not with overall cardiometabolic risk (Nettleton, Lutsey et al. 2009). In addition, findings from a national cohort study of 59,000 African American women demonstrated no association between ASB intake and diabetes risk, whereas the association between SSB and diabetes risk was positive, although of modest strength (Palmer et al. 2008).

Whether any association between ASB and obesity and elevated blood glucose would persist after adjusting for dieting practices and baseline health status, that is, reverse causality testing, remains an important question that was recently examined in detail by de Koning et al. (de Koning, Malik et al. 2011) using data from the Health Professionals Follow-Up Study. In this study, SSB and ASB both had positive associations with the risk of incident type 2 diabetes. However, after adjusting for dieting practices, baseline body mass index, and health status, the association was weakened and not no longer statistically significant for ASB, while the association remained robust for SSB. Thus, consistent with the findings form Project Eat for ASB and weight gain in youth described earlier (Vanselow, Pereira et al. 2009), it appears that the association between ASB and type 2 diabetes is likely an artifact of reverse causality, as those who are at higher risk for weight gain, obesity, and type 2 diabetes to begin with may be likely to increase ASB intake in order to attempt to reduce their risk. Indeed, recent findings from the CARDIA Study suggest that associations between reported intake of ASB and several risk factors for diabetes and cardiovascular disease may depend on whether the participants dietary pattern was described as Western or Prudent (Duffey, Steffen et al. 2012). However, the study did not adjust for intentional dieting for weight loss, and thus reverse causality remains likely.

Summary of artificially sweetened beverages

The epidemiologic and experimental studies on ASB and risk obesity and type 2 diabetes are lacking in rigor and consistency. Most studies have important limitations or were not able to address many sources of bias, especially reverse causality. The latter point is critical in observational studies because people attempting weight loss report more ASB consumption than those not trying to lose weight (Mozaffarian, Hao et al. 2011; Fowler, Williams et al. 2008; Vanselow, Pereira et al. 2009; de Koning, Malik et al. 2011). Although the hypothesis that ASB may stimulate appetite and lead to weight gain has become popular, it has not been supported by experimental human studies to date (Renwick and Molinary; Mattes and Popkin 2009). In fact, the evidence is suggesting the opposite, that obesity risk may be lower (weight loss or weight gain prevention) when ASB replace sugar-sweetened beverages in the diet (Tordoff and Alleva 1990; Raben, Vasilaras et al. 2002; Ebbeling, Feldman et al. 2006).

Prospective observational studies have revealed inconsistent findings on the association between ASB intake and risk for obesity (Ludwig et al. 2001; Schulze et al. 2004; Blum, Jacobsen et al. 2005; Fowler, Williams et al. 2008; Nettleton, Lutsey et al. 2009; Vanselow, Pereira et al. 2009) or cardiometabolic diseases including type 2 diabetes (Schulze et al. 2004; Dhingra, Sullivan et al. 2007; Lutsey, Steffen et al. 2008; Fung, Malik et al. 2009; Nettleton, Lutsey et al. 2009; de Koning, Malik et al. 2011). Importantly, with respect to reverse causality, two well-designed studies with repeated measures of diet and outcomes have demonstrated that any positive association between ASB and body weight or diabetes risk appears to be explained by reverse causality bias (de Koning, Malik et al. 2011; Vanselow, Pereira et al. 2009).

Due to the many limits of large epidemiologic studies, observational cohort studies are not likely to contribute to clear and consistent findings on this topic, although it is possible that the pooling of rich, high-quality data sets across large studies could help in clearing up some of the inconsistencies that remain in the literature. Randomized experimental studies may be particularly helpful, especially those that are relatively large and long term—at least several months in duration to allow ample study of caloric balance and body weight regulation, as well as possible changes in cardiometabolic risk factors. Studies should include diversity across age groups, gender, ethnicity, and other socioeconomic factors. Further, due to the hypothesis that ASB may perpetuate or reinforce a preference for sweet foods and drinks, studies should also examine the value of substituting water or other unsweetened beverages. The overall background habitual diet of the study participants must be measured well in observational or experimental studies, as well as physical activity and other potential confounding or modifying factors.

Coffee and T2D

Coffee has been a very important part of human culture for thousands of years, and is one of the richest sources of antioxidants in the diet (Natella and Scaccini 2012). The majority of coffee consumed is caffeinated. Recent epidemiological cohort studies have observed no consistent harm or benefit linked to intake of caffeine within the context of normal diets in the general population. However, possible metabolic effects of caffeine, such as its influence on fatty acid metabolism, metabolic rate, and other aspects of human performance continue to receive much attention. In any case, what has become quite clear in the literature is the lack of any robust association between caffeine intake and risk for T2D (Isogawa, Noda et al. 2003; Lane, Barkauskas et al. 2004; Salazar-Martinez, Willett et al. 2004; Graham, Sathasivam et al. 2001; Greer, Hudson et al. 2001). Therefore, the myriad minerals, antioxidants, and phytochemical compounds found in coffee beans may explain associations with diabetes risk.

Potential mechanisms

Figure 7.1 summarizes some of the theoretical mechanistic pathways through which coffee intake may impact diabetes risk.

Coffee appears to have powerful antioxidant properties (Natella, Nardini et al. 2002) that could potentially protect the pancreatic beta cell from oxidative stress or promote insulin sensitivity in the peripheral tissues, thereby delaying or preventing the onset of type 2 diabetes. A study of the Norwegian diet found coffee to contribute more antioxidants than any other dietary component (Svilaas, Sakhi et al. 2004). Unfortunately, typical nutritional epidemiologic data sources do not include the vast, although poorly understood, phytochemicals and other components of plant-based foods and beverages.

Nonetheless, short-term human and animal mechanistic studies have implicated chlorogenic acid (CGA), trigonelline, quinides, and magnesium in glucose metabolism. In animal studies, administration of trigonelline (Mishkinsky, Joseph et al. 1967) and CGA (Andrade-Cetto and

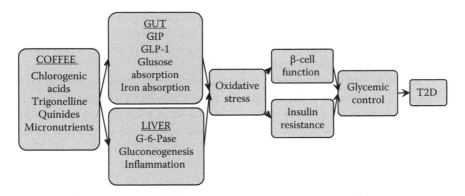

Figure 7.1 Theoretical casual model for effects of coffee on risk of T2D.

Wiedenfeld 2001; Rodriguez de Sotillo and Hadley 2002; Bassoli, Cassolla et al. 2008) improved postload glucose tolerance. In a randomized trial of adults with diabetes, administration of CGA resulted in significantly reduced postprandial plasma glucose levels (Herrera-Arellano, Aguilar-Santamaria et al. 2004) However, in healthy subjects, CGA and trigonelline only decreased glucose and insulin concentrations 15 minutes after a glucose load (van Dijk, Olthof et al. 2009). Moreover, some (Naismith, Akinyanju et al. 1970; Battram, Arthur et al. 2006) but not all (Johnston, Clifford et al. 2003; Louie, Atkinson et al. 2008; van Dijk, Olthof et al. 2009) human studies found decaffeinated coffee lowered postprandial glucose compared to placebo.

Coffee may affect postprandial glucose metabolism by inhibiting (Welsch, Lachance et al. 1989; McCarty 2005) or delaying absorption of glucose in the gut (Johnston, Clifford et al. 2003). Several human experimental studies have found that ingestion of decaffeinated coffee caused postprandial changes in GIP (Johnston, Clifford et al. 2003; Greenberg, Owen et al. 2010) and GLP-1 (Johnston, Clifford et al. 2003; Olthof, van Dijk et al. 2011)—gut hormones that are released in response to nutrient ingestion and responsible for 50% to 70% of insulin responsiveness (McCarty 2005). This suggests that coffee may shift glucose uptake from the proximal to more distal regions of the small intestine.

A specific polyphenol abundant in coffee, CGA, may also improve postprandial glucose via inhibition of glucose-6-phosphatase (G-6-Pase), an enzyme promoting lipid (Arion, Canfield et al. 1997; Bassoli, Cassolla et al. 2008; Henry-Vitrac, Ibarra et al. 2010). Another in vitro study found CGA specifically inhibited glucose-6-translocase, a component of the G-6-Pase system, thereby reducing both gluconeogenesis and glycogenolysis (Arion, Canfield et al. 1997). In addition to improving hepatic glucose output, CGA enhanced glucose uptake in skeletal muscle cells of mice through activation of AMP-activated protein kinase (Prabhakar and Doble

2009; Ong, Hsu et al. 2012). Moreover, in a cellular model, acute administration of quinidine, a polyphenol by-product of roasted CGA, increased
whole body insulin sensitivity through expression of the glucose transporter GLUT 4 (Shearer, Farah et al. 2003).

Another pathway whereby coffee may exert antidiabetic effects is
through iron chelation (Mascitelli, Pezzetta et al. 2007). Higher iron body
stores have been associated with an increased risk for T2D (Lee, Folsom
et al. 2004). CGA is a potent inhibitor of non-heme iron absorption when
consumed with the dietary source of iron (Fleming, Jacques et al. 1998).
Hurrell et al. found that the polyphenol content of a cup of coffee reduces
iron absorption from a test meal by 60% to 90% (Hurrell, Reddy et al. 1999).
Moreover, a one-cup per day increment in coffee consumption among
elderly participants in the Framingham Heart Study was associated with
a 1% lower serum ferritin concentration (Fleming, Jacques et al. 1998).

A recent review of the literature (Natella and Scaccini 2012) suggested that CGA, caffeic acid, and ferulic acid may also regulate the cellular processes that lead to inflammation. This hypothesis is supported
by observational (Homan and Mobarhan 2006; Williams, Fargnoli et al.
2008; Imatoh, Tanihara et al. 2011) and experimental (Kempf, Herder et
al. 2010; Wedick, Brennan et al. 2011) studies that have linked coffee to
higher insulin-sensitizing (Li, Shin et al. 2009) adiponectin concentrations
and lower levels of subclinical inflammatory markers, including fetuin-
A (Wedick, Brennan et al. 2011) and IL-18 (Kempf, Herder et al. 2010).
Improved adiponectin, IL-18, and fetuin-A levels have been associated
with lower T2D risk in observational studies (Thorand, Kolb et al. 2005; Ix,
Wassel et al. 2008; Li, Shin et al. 2009). Finally, in some (Esposito, Morisco
et al. 2003; Yoshida, Hayakawa et al. 2008; Kempf, Herder et al. 2010) but
not all studies (Mursu, Voutilainen et al. 2005), the antioxidant potential of
coffee-derived compounds have been linked to improved oxidative stress,
including higher 8-isoprostane levels, (Kempf, Herder et al. 2010) a marker
which has been inversely associated with T2D risk (Stephens, Khanolkar
et al. 2009).

Experimental evidence

Few intervention trials of coffee consumption and glucose homeostasis longer than one day have been conducted. The first intervention
study, which did not include a control group, found that 14 days of DC
intake reduced plasma glucose concentrations (Naismith, Akinyanju et
al. 1970). van Dam et al. analyzed a crossover coffee trial of 40 healthy,
caffeinated-coffee consuming (≥5 cups/day) adults and assigned them,
in random order, to 1-liter of coffee or abstention from coffee for 4 weeks
(van Dam, Pasman et al. 2004). The study that found 4 weeks of high

coffee consumption did not affect fasting glucose and increased fasting insulin concentrations.

Kempf et al. (Kempf, Herder et al. 2010) conducted a nonrandomized, three-stage clinical trial of 3 months (1 month per stage) that evaluated the effects of coffee on subclinical inflammation. Forty-seven nondiabetic coffee drinkers consumed no coffee for the first month, four cups of coffee/day for the second month, and eight cups of coffee/day for the third month. No effects were observed on measures of glucose metabolism, but higher coffee intake decreased the proinflammatory marker interleukin-18 (IL-18) and increased levels of adiponectin, HDL, and apolipoprotein A1 (Kempf, Herder et al. 2010). These favorable changes were more pronounced in insulin-resistant participants. Coffee intake also reduced the oxidative stress marker 8-isoprostane, which supports the antioxidant potential of coffee (Kempf, Herder et al. 2010).

In the longest trial on this topic to date, Wedick et al. randomized 45 healthy overweight volunteers, who were nonsmokers and caffeinated-coffee consumers, to five cups of CC, DC, or water per day for 8 weeks (Wedick, Brennan et al. 2011). While no changes in glucose homeostasis were observed, the study showed that coffee consumption may improve liver and adipocyte function through affecting the levels of ferritin-A and adiponectin, proteins associated with type 2 diabetes risk. The interventions in humans to date are modest, and they provide limited evidence that coffee intake may improve measures of glucose homeostasis and relevant biomarkers of risk over the short term.

Epidemiologic evidence

Epidemiologic studies reporting on hyperglycemia and insulin sensitivity, although fewer in number, are of particular interest as they provide insight into the key physiologic aspects of glucose metabolism affected by coffee consumption. A recent cross-sectional study found that coffee intake was associated with increased insulin sensitivity and reduced 2-hour postprandial glucose (i.e., 2-hour glucose) (Loopstra-Masters, Liese et al. 2011). This positive association between coffee intake and insulin sensitivity is consistent with Dutch (van Dam, Dekker et al. 2004), Swedish (Agardh, Carlsson et al. 2004; Arnlov, Vessby et al. 2004), and Asian (Rebello, Chen et al. 2011) studies. Consumption of decaffeinated coffee in particular was associated with improved 2-hour glucose and measures of β-cell function, including acute insulin response and proinsulin-to-peptide ratio. Some (Wu, Willett et al. 2005), but not all (Agardh, Carlsson et al. 2004; Arnlov, Vessby et al. 2004) human studies provide support for the hypothesis that decaffeinated coffee improves β-cell function. Nonetheless, results from these and other studies (Yamaji, Mizoue et al. 2004; Hamer, Witte et al.

2008) suggest that coffee consumption affects postprandial blood glucose more strongly than fasting glucose concentrations.

A prospective study from France supports the notion that the inverse association between coffee and diabetes is explained by coffee's effect on postprandial glucose metabolism (Sartorelli, Fagherazzi et al. 2010). They found that coffee consumed with the largest meal of the day explained the inverse association between coffee and diabetes in their study. The authors hypothesized that this association was due to coffee's ability to delay glucose absorption in the gut, but they could not rule out that the association was due to the iron-chelating effect of polyphenols in coffee.

Careful systematic reviews and meta-analyses on the topic of coffee, tea, and type 2 diabetes have indeed provided compelling evidence that, at least in prospective observational studies, coffee intake has a consistent protective, dose-response association with risk of T2D (van Dam and Hu 2005; Huxley, Lee et al. 2009). A recent meta-analysis by Huxley and colleagues included a synthesis of 18 studies and nearly a half million research subjects (Huxley, Lee et al. 2009). As shown in Figure 7.2, the findings for inverse (protective) associations between coffee and tea intake with risk of type 2 diabetes are astounding in their consistency, especially when one considers the breadth and diversity of the studies and the understandable measurement error in dietary intake as well as in the outcome assessment of most of the studies. Of 37 associations between coffee, tea, and diabetes risk estimated in this literature, 34 of them are inverse associations, most of those are statistically significant, three associations are clearly null, and none suggest a positive (adverse) association (Huxley, Lee et al. 2009).

Interestingly, the subset of studies that also presented findings for decaffeinated coffee suggest that the association is at least as strong, or stronger, than for regular coffee (Huxley, Lee et al. 2009). Therefore, it may be inferred that caffeine does not play a role in the protective association between coffee and risk of T2D. Indeed, in the Singapore Chinese Health Study, Odegaard et al. observed no association between caffeine intake and risk of T2D (Odegaard et al. 2008) and in the Iowa Women's Health Study Pereira et al. (Pereira, Parker et al. 2006) observed a considerably stronger inverse association between decaffeinated coffee intake and T2D risk than between caffeinated coffee and T2D risk. Unfortunately, there have been few experimental studies on this topic, and they are of short duration with a variety of inconsistencies and limitations. Relatively long-term, large, well-designed experimental studies on coffee, tea, and diabetes risk are needed.

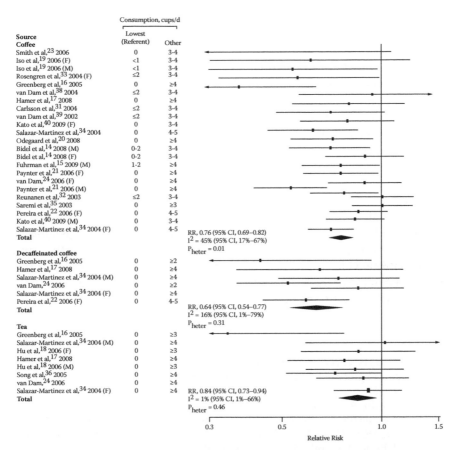

Figure 7.2 Association between coffee, decaffeinated coffee, and tea consumption and subsequent type 2 diabetes mellitus in published cohort studies (adjusted in all cases at least for age, sex, and body mass index). The studies are sorted by statistical size, defined by the inverse of the variance of the relative risk (RR). The center of each black square is propotional to the statistical size; and each horizontal line shows the 95% confidence interval (CI) for the estimate for each study. P_{heter} indicates P value for heterogeneity. (From Huxley, R., C. M. Lee et al. (2009). *Arch. Intern. Med.* **169**(22): 2053–2063.)

Summary of coffee

Over the past decade a prospective inverse association between coffee consumption and risk of type 2 diabetes has been consistently demonstrated in the epidemiologic literature. This association is quite strong and robust, perhaps more so than any other dietary factor that has been associated with type 2 diabetes risk to date. It appears to be independent of all known risk factors for type 2 diabetes, including body weight or obesity status. Interestingly, the possible list of casual agents in coffee does not include the caffeine. Individual studies as well as meta-analysis have shown that the association between coffee intake and risk of diabetes is at least as strong for consumption of decaffeinated coffee and it is for regular coffee. Furthermore, caffeine intake itself has not been consistently shown to be associated with risk of type 2 diabetes. Thus, the likely mechanisms of action include the many polyphenolic compounds and other phytochemicals and/or minerals found in coffee. Many of these individual components have been suggested through laboratory studies to have powerful antioxidant effects and also to play a role in the control of blood sugar through various pathways that may involve hormonal effects starting in the gut, or through effects on peripheral tissues including skeletal muscle, liver, or the pancreas. However, a possible direct causal effect of coffee on risk of diabetes cannot be established without sufficient experimental evidence on this topic. Such studies must include human subjects at risk for type 2 diabetes, valid measures of mechanisms of action, and well-controlled clinical trials that are designed to firmly test efficacy. It is likely that many of the answers to these various pieces of the causal chain will be addressed by scientists in the near future.

References

Agardh, E. E., S. Carlsson et al. (2004). "Coffee consumption, type 2 diabetes and impaired glucose tolerance in Swedish men and women." *J Intern Med* **255**(6): 645–652.

Andrade-Cetto, A. and H. Wiedenfeld (2001). "Hypoglycemic effect of Cecropia obtusifolia on streptozotocin diabetic rats." *J Ethnopharmacol* **78**(2–3): 145–149.

Arion, W. J., W. K. Canfield et al. (1997). "Chlorogenic acid and hydroxynitrobenzaldehyde: New inhibitors of hepatic glucose 6-phosphatase." *Arch Biochem Biophys* **339**(2): 315–322.

Arnlov, J., B. Vessby et al. (2004). "Coffee consumption and insulin sensitivity." *JAMA* **291**(10): 1199–1201.

Bassoli, B. K., P. Cassolla et al. (2008). "Chlorogenic acid reduces the plasma glucose peak in the oral glucose tolerance test: Effects on hepatic glucose release and glycaemia." *Cell Biochem Funct* **26**(3): 320–328.

Battram, D. S., R. Arthur et al. (2006). "The glucose intolerance induced by caffeinated coffee ingestion is less pronounced than that due to alkaloid caffeine in men." *J Nutr* **136**(5): 1276–1280.

Berkey, C. S., H. R. Rockett, A. E. Field, M. W. Gillman, and G. A. Colditz (2004). "Sugar-added beverages and adolescent weight change." *Obes Res* **12**: 778–788.

Bleich, S. N., Y. C. Wang et al. (2009). "Increasing consumption of sugar-sweetened beverages among US adults: 1988–1994 to 1999–2004." *Am J Clin Nutr* **89**(1): 372–381.

Blum, J. W., D. J. Jacobsen et al. (2005). "Beverage consumption patterns in elementary school aged children across a two-year period." *J Am Coll Nutr* **24**(2): 93–98.

Brown, R. J., M. Walter, and K. I. Rother (2009). "Ingestion of diet soda before a glucose load augments glucagon-like peptide-1 secretion." *Diabetes Care* **32**(12): 2184–2186.

Choi, J. W., E. S. Ford, X. Gao, and H. K. Choi (2008). "Sugar-sweetened soft drinks, diet soft drinks, and serum uric acid level: The Third National Health and Nutrition Examination Survey." *Arthritis Rheum* **15**(59): 109–116.

de Koning, L., V. S. Malik et al. (2011). "Sugar-sweetened and artificially sweetened beverage consumption and risk of type 2 diabetes in men." *Am J Clin Nutr* **93**(6): 1321–1327.

Dhingra, R., L. Sullivan et al. (2007). "Soft drink consumption and risk of developing cardiometabolic risk Factors and the metabolic syndrome in middle-aged adults in the community." *Circulation* **116**(5): 480–488.

DiMeglio, D. P. and R. D. Mattes (2000). "Liquid versus solid carbohydrate: Effects on food intake and body weight." *Int J Obes Relat Metab Disord* **24**(6): 794–800.

Duffey, K. J., L. M. Steffen et al. (2012). "Dietary patterns matter: Diet beverages and cardiometabolic risks in the longitudinal Coronary Artery Risk Development in Young Adults (CARDIA) Study." *Am J Clin Nutr* **95**(4): 909–915.

Ebbeling, C. B., H. A. Feldman et al. (2006). "Effects of decreasing sugar-sweetened beverage consumption on body weight in adolescents: A randomized, controlled pilot study." *Pediatrics* **117**(3): 673–680.

Esposito, F., F. Morisco et al. (2003). "Moderate coffee consumption increases plasma glutathione but not homocysteine in healthy subjects." *Aliment Pharmacol Ther* **17**(4): 595–601.

Field, A. E., S. B. Austin et al. (2003). "Relation between dieting and weight change among preadolescents and adolescents." *Pediatrics* **112**(4): 900–906.

Fleming, D. J., P. F. Jacques et al. (1998). "Dietary determinants of iron stores in a free-living elderly population: The Framingham Heart Study." *Am J Clin Nutr* **67**(4): 722–733.

Ford, H. E., Peters V, Martin NM, Sleeth ML, Ghatei MA, Frost GS, Bloom SR (2011). "Effects of oral ingestion of sucralose on gut hormone response and appetite in healthy normal-weight subjects." *Eur J Clin Nutr* **65**: 508–513.

Fowler, S. P., K. Williams et al. (2008). "Fueling the obesity epidemic? Artificially sweetened beverage use and long-term weight gain." *Obesity (Silver Spring)* **16**(8): 1894–1900.

French, S. A., B. H. Lin et al. (2003). "National trends in soft drink consumption among children and adolescents age 6 to 17 years: Prevalence, amounts, and sources, 1977/1978 to 1994/1998." *J Am Diet Assoc* **103**(10): 1326–1331.

Fung, T. T., V. Malik et al. (2009). "Sweetened beverage consumption and risk of coronary heart disease in women." *Am J Clin Nutr* **89**(4): 1037–1042.

Graham, T. E., P. Sathasivam et al. (2001). "Caffeine ingestion elevates plasma insulin response in humans during an oral glucose tolerance test." *Can J Physiol Pharmacol* **79**(7): 559–565.

Greenberg, J. A., D. R. Owen et al. (2010). "Decaffeinated coffee and glucose metabolism in young men." *Diabetes Care* **33**(2): 278–280.

Greer, F., R. Hudson et al. (2001). "Caffeine ingestion decreases glucose disposal during a hyperinsulinemic-euglycemic clamp in sedentary humans." *Diabetes* **50**(10): 2349–2354.

Hamer, M., D. R. Witte et al. (2008). "Prospective study of coffee and tea consumption in relation to risk of type 2 diabetes mellitus among men and women: The Whitehall II study." *Br J Nutr* **100**(5): 1046–1053.

Harnack, L., J. Stang et al. (1999). "Soft drink consumption among US children and adolescents: Nutritional consequences." *J Am Diet Assoc* **99**(4): 436–441.

Henry-Vitrac, C., A. Ibarra et al. (2010). "Contribution of chlorogenic acids to the inhibition of human hepatic glucose-6-phosphatase activity in vitro by Svetol, a standardized decaffeinated green coffee extract." *J Agric Food Chem* **58**(7): 4141–4144.

Herrera-Arellano, A., L. Aguilar-Santamaria et al. (2004). "Clinical trial of Cecropia obtusifolia and Marrubium vulgare leaf extracts on blood glucose and serum lipids in type 2 diabetics." *Phytomedicine* **11**(7–8): 561–566.

Homan, D. J. and S. Mobarhan (2006). "Coffee: Good, bad, or just fun? A critical review of coffee's effects on liver enzymes." *Nutr Rev* **64**(1): 43–46.

Hurrell, R. F., M. Reddy et al. (1999). "Inhibition of non-haem iron absorption in man by polyphenolic-containing beverages." *Br J Nutr* **81**(4): 289–295.

Huxley, R., C. M. Lee et al. (2009). "Coffee, decaffeinated coffee, and tea consumption in relation to incident type 2 diabetes mellitus: A systematic review with meta-analysis." *Arch Intern Med* **169**(22): 2053–2063.

Imatoh, T., S. Tanihara et al. (2011). "Coffee consumption but not green tea consumption is associated with adiponectin levels in Japanese males." *Eur J Nutr* **50**(4): 279–284.

Isogawa, A., M. Noda et al. (2003). "Coffee consumption and risk of type 2 diabetes mellitus." *Lancet* **361**(9358): 703–704.

Ix, J. H., C. L. Wassel et al. (2008). "Fetuin-A and incident diabetes mellitus in older persons." *JAMA* **300**(2): 182–188.

James, J., P. Thomas et al. (2004). "Preventing childhood obesity by reducing consumption of carbonated drinks: Cluster randomised controlled trial." *BMJ* **328**(7450): 1237.

Jang, H. J., Z. Kokrashvili, M. J. Theodorakis, O. D. Carlson, B. J. Kim, J. Zhou, H. H. Kim, X. Xu, S. L. Chan, M. Juhaszova, M. Bernier, B. Mosinger, R. F. Margolskee, and J. M. Egan (2007). "Gut-expressed gustducin and taste receptors regulate secretion of glucagon-like peptide-1." *Proc Natl.*

Johnston, K. L., M. N. Clifford et al. (2003). "Coffee acutely modifies gastrointestinal hormone secretion and glucose tolerance in humans: Glycemic effects of chlorogenic acid and caffeine." *Am J Clin Nutr* **78**(4): 728–733.

Kempf, K., C. Herder et al. (2010). "Effects of coffee consumption on subclinical inflammation and other risk factors for type 2 diabetes: A clinical trial." *Am J Clin Nutr* **91**(4): 950–957.

Lane, J. D., C. E. Barkauskas et al. (2004). "Caffeine impairs glucose metabolism in type 2 diabetes." *Diabetes Care* **27**(8): 2047–2048.

Lee, D. H., A. R. Folsom et al. (2004). "Dietary iron intake and Type 2 diabetes incidence in postmenopausal women: The Iowa Women's Health Study." *Diabetologia* **47**(2): 185–194.

Li, S., H. J. Shin et al. (2009). "Adiponectin levels and risk of type 2 diabetes: A systematic review and meta-analysis." *JAMA* **302**(2): 179–188.

Loopstra-Masters, R. C., A. D. Liese et al. (2011). "Associations between the intake of caffeinated and decaffeinated coffee and measures of insulin sensitivity and beta cell function." *Diabetologia* **54**(2): 320–328.

Louie, J. C., F. Atkinson et al. (2008). "Delayed effects of coffee, tea and sucrose on postprandial glycemia in lean, young, healthy adults." *Asia Pac J Clin Nutr* **17**(4): 657–662.

Ludwig, D. S. (2009). "Artificially sweetened beverages: Cause for concern." *JAMA* **302**(22): 2477–2478.

Ludwig, D. S., K. E. Peterson, and S. L. Gortmaker (2001). "Relation between consumption of sugar-sweetened drinks and childhood obesity: A prospective, observational analysis." *Lancet* **357**: 505–508.

Lutsey, P. L., L. M. Steffen et al. (2008). "Dietary intake and the development of the metabolic syndrome: The Atherosclerosis Risk in Communities study." *Circulation* **117**(6): 754–761.

Ma, J., M. Bellon, J. M. Wishart, R. Young, L. A. Blackshaw, K. L. Jones, M. Horowitz, and C. K. Rayner (2009). "Effect of the artificial sweetener, sucralose, on gastric emptying and incretin hormone release in healthy subjects." *Am J Physiol Gastrointest Liver Physiol* **296**(4): 735–739.

Mackenzie., T., B. Brooks, and G. O'Connor (2006). "Beverage intake, diabetes, and glucose control of adults in America." *Ann Epidemiol* **16**(9): 688–691.

Maersk, M., A. Belza et al. (2012). "Sucrose-sweetened beverages increase fat storage in the liver, muscle, and visceral fat depot: A 6-mo randomized intervention study." *Am J Clin Nutr* **95**(2): 283–289.

Mascitelli, L., F. Pezzetta et al. (2007). "Inhibition of iron absorption by coffee and the reduced risk of type 2 diabetes mellitus." *Arch Intern Med* **167**(2): 204–205; author reply 205.

Mattes, R. D. and B. M. Popkin (2009). "Nonnutritive sweetener consumption in humans: Effects on appetite and food intake and their putative mechanisms." *Am J Clin Nutr* **89**(1): 1–14.

McCarty, M. F. (2005). "A chlorogenic acid-induced increase in GLP-1 production may mediate the impact of heavy coffee consumption on diabetes risk." *Med Hypotheses* **64**(4): 848–853.

Mishkinsky, J., B. Joseph et al. (1967). "Hypoglycaemic effect of trigonelline." *Lancet* **2**(7529): 1311–1312.

Mozaffarian, D., T. Hao et al. (2011). "Changes in diet and lifestyle and long-term weight gain in women and men." *N Engl J Med* **364**(25): 2392–2404.

Mursu, J., S. Voutilainen et al. (2005). "The effects of coffee consumption on lipid peroxidation and plasma total homocysteine concentrations: A clinical trial." *Free Radic Biol Med* **38**(4): 527–534.

Naismith, D. J., P. A. Akinyanju et al. (1970). "The effect, in volunteers, of coffee and decaffeinated coffee on blood glucose, insulin, plasma lipids and some factors involved in blood clotting." *Nutr Metab* **12**(3): 144–151.

Natella, F., M. Nardini et al. (2002). "Coffee drinking influences plasma antioxidant capacity in humans." *J Agric Food Chem* **50**(21): 6211–6216.

Natella, F., Scaccini, C. (2012). "Role of coffee in modulation of diabetes risk." *Nutr Rev* **70**(4): 207–217.

Nelson, G., M. A. Hoon, J. Chandrashekar, Y. Zhang, N. J. Ryba, and C. S. Zuker (2001). "Mammalian sweet taste receptors." *Cell* **106**(3): 381–390.

Nettleton, J. A., P. L. Lutsey et al. (2009). "Diet soda intake and risk of incident metabolic syndrome and type 2 diabetes in the Multi-Ethnic Study of Atherosclerosis (MESA)." *Diabetes Care* **32**(4): 688–694.

Neumark-Sztainer, D., M. Wall et al. (2006). "Obesity, disordered eating, and eating disorders in a longitudinal study of adolescents: How do dieters fare 5 years later?" *J Am Diet Assoc* **106**(4): 559–568.

Odegaard, A. O., M. A. Pereira, W, P. Koh, K. Arakawa, H. P. Lee, and M. C. Yu (2008). "Coffee, tea and incident type 2 diabetes: The Singapore Chinese Health Study." *Am J Clin Nutr* **88**(4): 979–985.

Olthof, M. R., A. E. van Dijk et al. (2011). "Acute effects of decaffeinated coffee and the major coffee components chlorogenic acid and trigonelline on incretin hormones." *Nutr Metab (Lond)* **8**: 10.

Ong, K. W., A. Hsu et al. (2012). "Chlorogenic acid stimulates glucose transport in skeletal muscle via AMPK activation: A contributor to the beneficial effects of coffee on diabetes." *PLoS One* **7**(3): e32718.

Palmer, J., Boggs, DA., Krishnan, S. et al. (2008). "Sugar-sweetened beverages and incidence of type 2 diabetes mellitus in african american women." *Arch Intern Med* **168**(14): 1487–1492.

Pereira, M. A., E. D. Parker et al. (2006). "Coffee consumption and risk of type 2 diabetes mellitus: An 11-year prospective study of 28 812 postmenopausal women." *Arch Intern Med* **166**(12): 1311–1316.

Popkin, B. M. (2010). "Patterns of beverage use across the lifecycle." *Physiol Behav* **100**(1): 4–9.

Prabhakar, P. K. and M. Doble (2009). "Synergistic effect of phytochemicals in combination with hypoglycemic drugs on glucose uptake in myotubes." *Phytomedicine* **16**(12): 1119–1126.

Raben, A. (2002). "Should obese patients be counselled to follow a low-glycaemic index diet? No." *Obes Rev* **3**(4): 245–256.

Raben, A., T. H. Vasilaras et al. (2002). "Sucrose compared with artificial sweeteners: Different effects on ad libitum food intake and body weight after 10 wk of supplementation in overweight subjects." *Am J Clin Nutr* **76**(4): 721–729.

Rebello, S. A., C. H. Chen et al. (2011). "Coffee and tea consumption in relation to inflammation and basal glucose metabolism in a multi-ethnic Asian population: A cross-sectional study." *Nutr J* **10**: 61.

Renwick, A. G. and S. V. Molinary "Sweet-taste receptors, low-energy sweeteners, glucose absorption and insulin release." *Br J Nutr* **104**(10): 1415–1420.

Rodriguez de Sotillo, D. V. and M. Hadley (2002). "Chlorogenic acid modifies plasma and liver concentrations of: Cholesterol, triacylglycerol, and minerals in (fa/fa) Zucker rats." *J Nutr Biochem* **13**(12): 717–726.

Salazar-Martinez, E., W. C. Willett et al. (2004). "Coffee consumption and risk for type 2 diabetes mellitus." *Ann Intern Med* **140**(1): 1–8.

Sartorelli, D. S., G. Fagherazzi et al. (2010). "Differential effects of coffee on the risk of type 2 diabetes according to meal consumption in a French cohort of women: The E3N/EPIC cohort study." *Am J Clin Nutr* **91**(4): 1002–1012.

Schulze, M. B., J. E. Manson, D. S. Ludwig, G. A. Colditz, M. J. Stampfer, W. C. Willett, and F. B. Hu (2004). "Sugar-sweetened beverages, weight gain, and incidence of type 2 diabetes in young and middle-aged women." *JAMA* **292**: 927–934.

Shearer, J., A. Farah et al. (2003). "Quinides of roasted coffee enhance insulin action in conscious rats." *J Nutr* **133**(11): 3529–3532.

Sichieri, R., A. Paula Trotte et al. (2009). "School randomised trial on prevention of excessive weight gain by discouraging students from drinking sodas." *Public Health Nutr* **12**(2): 197–202.

Smolin, L., Benevenga, N. Accumulation of homocysteinemia in vitamin B6 deficiency. *J Nutr* 1982; **112**: 1264–72.

Steinert, R. E., F. Frey, A. Töpfer, J. Drewe, and C. Beglinger (2011). "Effects of carbohydrate sugars and artificial sweeteners on appetite and the secretion of gastrointestinal satiety peptides." *Br J Nutr* **105**(9): 1320–1328.

Stephens, J. W., M. P. Khanolkar et al. (2009). "The biological relevance and measurement of plasma markers of oxidative stress in diabetes and cardiovascular disease." *Atherosclerosis* **202**(2): 321–329.

Stice, E., R. P. Cameron et al. (1999). "Naturalistic weight-reduction efforts prospectively predict growth in relative weight and onset of obesity among female adolescents." *J Consult Clin Psychol* **67**(6): 967–974.

Stice, E., K. Presnell et al. (2005). "Psychological and behavioral risk factors for obesity onset in adolescent girls: A prospective study." *J Consult Clin Psychol* **73**(2): 195–202.

Striegel-Moore, R. H., D. Thompson et al. (2006). "Correlates of beverage intake in adolescent girls: The National Heart, Lung, and Blood Institute Growth and Health Study." *J Pediatr* **148**(2): 183–187.

Svilaas, A., A. K. Sakhi et al. (2004). "Intakes of antioxidants in coffee, wine, and vegetables are correlated with plasma carotenoids in humans." *J Nutr* **134**(3): 562–567.

Swithers, S. E., A. A. Martin, and T. L. Davidson (2010). "High-intensity sweeteners and energy balance." *Physiol Behav* **100**(1): 55–62.

Tate, D. F., G. Turner-McGrievy et al. (2012). "Replacing caloric beverages with water or diet beverages for weight loss in adults: Main results of the Choose Healthy Options Consciously Everyday (CHOICE) randomized clinical trial." *Am J Clin Nutr* **95**(3): 555–563.

Thorand, B., H. Kolb et al. (2005). "Elevated levels of interleukin-18 predict the development of type 2 diabetes: Results from the MONICA/KORA Augsburg Study, 1984–2002." *Diabetes* **54**(10): 2932–2938.

Tordoff, M. G. and A. M. Alleva (1990). "Effect of drinking soda sweetened with aspartame or high-fructose corn syrup on food intake and body weight." *Am J Clin Nutr* **51**(6): 963–969.

van Dam, R. M., J. M. Dekker et al. (2004). "Coffee consumption and incidence of impaired fasting glucose, impaired glucose tolerance, and type 2 diabetes: The Hoorn Study." *Diabetologia* **47**(12): 2152–2159.

van Dam, R. M. and F. B. Hu (2005). "Coffee consumption and risk of type 2 diabetes: A systematic review." *JAMA* **294**(1): 97–104.

van Dam, R. M., W. J. Pasman et al. (2004). "Effects of coffee consumption on fasting blood glucose and insulin concentrations: Randomized controlled trials in healthy volunteers." *Diabetes Care* **27**(12): 2990–2992.

van Dijk, A. E., M. R. Olthof et al. (2009). "Acute effects of decaffeinated coffee and the major coffee components chlorogenic acid and trigonelline on glucose tolerance." *Diabetes Care* **32**(6): 1023–1025.

Vanselow, M. S., M. A. Pereira et al. (2009). "Adolescent beverage habits and changes in weight over time: Findings from Project EAT." *Am J Clin Nutr* **90**(6): 1489–1495.

Wedick, N. M., A. M. Brennan et al. (2011). "Effects of caffeinated and decaffeinated coffee on biological risk factors for type 2 diabetes: A randomized controlled trial." *Nutr J* **10**: 93.

Welsch, C. A., P. A. Lachance et al. (1989). "Dietary phenolic compounds: Inhibition of Na+-dependent D-glucose uptake in rat intestinal brush border membrane vesicles." *J Nutr* **119**(11): 1698–1704.

Williams, C. J., J. L. Fargnoli et al. (2008). "Coffee consumption is associated with higher plasma adiponectin concentrations in women with or without type 2 diabetes: A prospective cohort study." *Diabetes Care* **31**(3): 504–507.

Wu, T., W. C. Willett et al. (2005). "Caffeinated coffee, decaffeinated coffee, and caffeine in relation to plasma C-peptide levels, a marker of insulin secretion, in U.S. women." *Diabetes Care* **28**(6): 1390–1396.

Wu, T., B. R. Zhao, M. J. Bound, H. L. Checklin, M. Bellon, T. J. Little, R. L. Young, K. L. Jones, M. Horowitz, and C. K. Rayner (2012). "Effects of different sweet preloads on incretin hormone secretion, gastric emptying, and postprandial glycemia in healthy humans." *Am J Clin Nutr* **95**(1): 78–83.

Yamaji, T., T. Mizoue et al. (2004). "Coffee consumption and glucose tolerance status in middle-aged Japanese men." *Diabetologia* **47**(12): 2145–2151.

Yen, S. T. and B.-H. Lin (2002). "Beverage consumption among US children and adolescents: Full-information and quasi maximum-likelihood estimation of a censored system." *Eur Rev Agric Economics* **29**(1): 85–103.

Yoshida, Y., M. Hayakawa et al. (2008). "Evaluation of the antioxidant effects of coffee and its components using the biomarkers hydroxyoctadecadienoic acid and isoprostane." *J Oleo Sci* **57**(12): 691–697.

Summary and directions for future research

Advancing the science on the role of nutrition in the etiology and prevention of type 2 diabetes will continue to primarily focus on carbohydrates, as emphasized in Chapter 2 of this text. Carbohydrates are the only nutrient that directly, acutely, and dramatically influence blood sugar, and carbohydrate intake has not only steadily increased over the past 50 years, but the quality of carbohydrate-based foods has appeared to decline when measured by processing, nutrient, and fiber density. There is no better example than sugar-sweetened beverages, which are consumed in higher quantities among youth in the United States than any other beverage including milk, and which are responsible for most of the added sugars in the American diet. The notion that carbohydrates are homogenous in their impact on health, either beneficial or harmful, is dogma of the past. Foods that are rich in carbohydrates vary wildly in their acute impact on blood sugar and insulin, and their chronic impact on health. Perhaps the most striking development in this area has been the emergence of consistent scientific evidence from observational studies on the association between sugar-sweetened beverages and risk of type 2 diabetes. However, in order to further our understanding of these associations, including the identification of the biological mechanisms, well-designed experimental studies are needed. While more science on the type and amounts of carbohydrates is needed, and especially in the context of experimentations, it makes sense to propose public health messages that focus on improving the density of fiber and micronutrients in the diet, and reducing the intake of foods that have added sugars and other highly processed ingredients.

Dietary fats and proteins, covered in Chapters 3 and 4, play essential and critical roles in human biological function; however, the role of different fatty acid and amino acid classes in the etiology and prevention of type 2 diabetes has some general direction but remains inconclusive. As for the other macronutrients, fatty acids and proteins, while not having

213

a direct effect on blood sugar per se, their effects through the gut and through more chronic systemic effects on peripheral insulin sensitivity and pancreatic beta-cell function continues to be an important area of research. Much remains to be discovered in the areas of protein and fatty acids and the risk of type 2 diabetes. Inconsistent results across fatty acid types and amino acid types with type 2 diabetes underlines the need to continue to carefully study the topic, update related study methods, analytical approaches, and creatively examine the subject matter. It is imperative that observational studies conduct analyses and interpret results in the spectrum of the overall dietary pattern, so the fatty acid and protein intake has some context with respect to specific types and qualities of foods and beverages in appropriate cultural contexts.

In terms of micronutrients (Chapter 5), including minerals, vitamins, and related "phytochemicals" that may have anti-inflammatory, antioxidant, and insulin-sensitizing properties, considerable uncertainty exists regarding specific mechanisms of actions and therefore efficacy and potential for public health implications. Current epidemiologic and clinical data cannot provide definitive answers regarding micronutrients in the primary prevention of type 2 diabetes due to the lack of long-term, large-scale randomized clinical trials. Findings from such trials are needed to move forward with more concrete scientific information for public health recommendations on specific dietary components in the prevention of type 2 diabetes.

The study of overall dietary patterns (covered in Chapter 6) in relation to chronic disease risk has the most potential to advance the science of diet and health and support public health messages and policies. Using modern epidemiological and statistical methods, the study of overall dietary patterns capitalizes on unique cultural aspects of total dietary intake, and on the overlapping and synergistic impact of dietary effects across the spectrum of foods and beverages consumed in the population. The literature on dietary patterns and type 2 diabetes risk carefully distilled in Chapter 6 can be reliably translated into general recommendations to consume a diet emphasizing vegetables, fruits, legumes, whole grains, nuts, and including (not in excess) dairy, varieties of seafood, unprocessed poultry, red meat and oils from fruits/nuts/seeds (e.g., olive, canola). On the other hand, items to limit in the diet, due to their potential to increase diabetes risk include sweetened foods and beverages, processed grains, cured meats, fatty meats, and deep-fried foods. The evidence to support these recommendations is consistent across different populations with different geographical, political, demographic, socioeconomic, and ethnic/racial characteristics.

While the epidemiologic evidence on sugar-sweetened beverages and risk of type 2 diabetes is robust and consistent, the epidemiologic and experimental studies on artificially sweetened beverages (ASB) and risk of type 2 diabetes is lacking in rigor and consistency, as explained in Chapter 7. Most studies have a variety of limitations and were not able to address many potential biases, especially reverse causality—those attempting weight loss report more ASB consumption than those not attempting weight loss. Indeed, the scientific evidence is suggesting that obesity risk may be lower (weight loss or weight gain prevention) when ASB replace sugar-sweetened beverages in the diet. Future experimental studies should include diversity across age groups, gender, ethnicity, and other socioeconomic factors.

Observational evidence accumulated over the past decade has consistently demonstrated a strong, robust association between coffee consumption and risk of type 2 diabetes (Chapter 7). In fact, this association appears to be stronger and more consistent than any other dietary factor that has been associated with type 2 diabetes risk to date. Importantly, the association between coffee consumption and risk of type 2 diabetes appears to be independent of all known risk factors for type 2 diabetes, including body weight or obesity status. Interestingly, caffeine does not appear to explain the association between coffee intake and diabetes risk. The suspected mechanisms of action thus include the many polyphenolic compounds and other phytochemicals and/or minerals in coffee, which may have important antioxidant effects or also play a role in glycemic control through hormonal effects via the gut or through effects on peripheral tissues (skeletal muscle, liver, or pancreas). Future studies on this topic must include human subjects at risk for type 2 diabetes and valid measures of possible mechanistic pathways.

In closing, it is still useful to use the criteria to evaluate causality introduced by Sir Austin Bradford Hill in 1965. Hill's "criteria for causation" continue to be a valuable guide when either setting out on a research endeavor, or when synthesizing the literature to evaluate the scientific evidence on a specific topic. With respect to the role of dietary composition and risk for type 2 diabetes, there is considerable evidence in most major areas of the dietary spectrum to satisfy Hill's criteria of causation: (1) strength of association, (2) consistency, (3) specificity, (4) temporality, (5) biological gradient, (6) coherence, (7) experimentation, and (8) analogy. The criteria of "experimentation" remains the area with the most potential to further our understanding of efficacy and effectiveness on the role of nutrition and dietary patterns in the prevention of type 2 diabetes.

Index

Milton Keynes UK
Ingram Content Group UK Ltd.
UKHW020313111024
449327UK00040B/756